T0226837

Sporting Injuries to the Foot & Ankle

Editor

JAMES D.F. CALDER

FOOT AND ANKLE CLINICS

www.foot.theclinics.com

Consulting Editor
MARK S. MYERSON

June 2013 • Volume 18 • Number 2

ELSEVIER

1600 John F. Kennedy Boulevard • Suite 1800 • Philadelphia, Pennsylvania, 19103-2899

http://www.theclinics.com

FOOT AND ANKLE CLINICS Volume 18, Number 2
June 2013 ISSN 1083-7515, ISBN-13: 978-1-4557-7089-2

Editor: Jennifer Flynn-Briggs

Foot and Ankle Clinics (ISSN 1083-7515) is published quarterly by Elsevier, Inc., 360 Park Avenue South, New York, NY 10010-1710. Months of issue are March, June, September, and December. Periodicals postage paid at New York, NY, and additional mailing offices. Subscription price per year is $299.00 (US individuals), $401.00 (US institutions), $148.00 (US students), $341.00 (Canadian individuals), $473.00 (Canadian institutions), $204.00 (Canadian students), $439.00 (foreign individuals), $473.00 (foreign institutions), and $204.00 (foreign students). To receive student/resident rate, orders must be accompanied by name of affiliated institution, date of term, and the *signature* of program/residency coordinator on institution letterhead. Orders will be billed at individual rate until proof of status is received. Foreign air speed delivery is included in all *Clinics* subscription prices. All prices are subject to change without notice. **POSTMASTER:** Send address changes to *Foot and Ankle Clinics*, Elsevier Health Sciences Division, Subscription Customer Service, 3251 Riverport Lane, Maryland Heights, MO 63043. **Customer Service: 1-800-654-2452 (US and Canada). From outside of the United States and Canada, call 314-447-8871. Fax: 314-447-8029. E-mail: JournalsCustomerService-usa@ elsevier.com (for print support); JournalsOnlineSupport-usa@elsevier.com (for online support).**

Reprints. For copies of 100 or more, of articles in this publication, please contact the Commercial Reprints Department, Elsevier Inc., 360 Park Avenue South, New York, NY 10010-1710. Tel.: 212-633-3812; Fax: 212-462-1935; E-mail: reprints@elsevier.com.

Printed and bound by CPI Group (UK) Ltd, Croydon, CR0 4YY

Transferred to digital print 2012

Contributors

CONSULTING EDITOR

MARK S. MYERSON, MD
Director, The Institute for Foot and Ankle Reconstruction, Mercy Medical Center, Baltimore, Maryland

EDITOR

JAMES D.F. CALDER, TD, MD, FRCS(Tr & Orth), FFSEM(UK)
Consultant Orthopedic Surgeon, Chelsea and Westminster Hospital, London, United Kingdom; Fortius Clinic, London, United Kingdom

AUTHORS

BENJAMIN C. CAESAR, MD, MBBS, FRCS Ed (Orth), FRCS
Diploma Sport and Exercise Medicine, Locum Consultant Orthopaedic Surgeon, Chelsea and Westminister Hospital, London, United Kingdom

JAMES D.F. CALDER, TD, MD, FRCS(Tr & Orth), FFSEM(UK)
Consultant Orthopaedic Surgeon, Chelsea and Westminster Hospital; Fortius Clinic, London, United Kingdom

VINCENZO DENARO, MD
Professor of Orthopaedic and Trauma Surgery, Department of Orthopaedic and Trauma Surgery, Campus Bio-Medico University, Trigoria; Centro Integrato di Ricerca (CIR), Campus Bio-Medico University, Rome, Italy

RUPINDERBIR SINGH DEOL, MSc, DIC, FRCS(Tr&Orth)
Consultant Orthopaedic Surgeon, Lister/QEII Hospitals, East and North Herts NHS Trust, Stevenage, Hertfordshire, United Kingdom

KYRIACOS I. ELEFTHERIOU, MD, FRCS(Tr & Orth)
Specialist Registrar, Department of Trauma and Orthopaedics, St Mary's Hospital, London, United Kingdom

ROBIN ELLIOT, MA, FRCS(Tr&Orth)
Consultant Orthopaedic Surgeon, Hampshire Hospitals NHS Trust, Basingstoke, Hampshire, United Kingdom

BRYAN ENGLISH, MB ChB, FFSEM
Consultant Physician in Sports and Exercise Medicine, The Fortius Clinic, London, United Kingdom

AJIT GARDE, FRCSOrth
Associate Specialist in Orthopaedic Surgery, Northampton General Hospital, Northampton, United Kingdom

LOUISE GARTNER, MBBS, MRCP, FRCR
Consultant Radiologist, Department of Radiology, National University Hospital,
Singapore, Republic of Singapore

ABHIJIT GUHA, FRCS(Tr & Orth)
Foot and Ankle Fellow, Department of Orthopaedics, Avon Orthopaedic Centre,
Southmead Hospital, Bristol, United Kingdom

STEPHANE GUILLO, MD
Centre for Orthopaedic Sports Surgery, Bordeaux-Mérignac, France

STEVE HEPPLE, MBChB, FRCS(Tr & Orth)
Consultant Orthopaedic Surgeon, Department of Orthopaedics, Foot Avon Orthopaedic
Centre, Southmead Hospital, Bristol, United Kingdom

IAIN T. JAMES, PhD
Senior Lecturer, Centre for Sports Surface Technology, Cranfield University; Presently:
Technical Director, TGMS Ltd, Cranfield Innovation Centre, Cranfield, United Kingdom

GINO M.M.J. KERKHOFFS, MD, PhD
Orthopedic Surgeon, Department of Orthopedic Surgery, Orthopedic Research Center
Amsterdam, Academic Medical Center, Amsterdam, The Netherlands

UMILE GIUSEPPE LONGO, MD, MSc, PhD
Specialist in Orthopaedic and Trauma Surgery, Department of Orthopaedic and Trauma
Surgery, Campus Bio-Medico University, Trigoria; Centro Integrato di Ricerca (CIR),
Campus Bio-Medico University, Rome, Italy

NICOLA MAFFULLI, MD, MS, PhD, FRCS(Orth)
Professor of Orthopaedic and Trauma Surgery, Centre for Sports and Exercise Medicine,
Barts and The London School of Medicine and Dentistry, Mile End Hospital, London,
England

MAY FONG MAK, MBChB, MRCS, MMed Ortho
Orthopaedic Registrar, Department of Orthopaedics, Khoo Teck Puat Hospital,
Singapore, Republic of Singapore

GRAHAM A. MCCOLLUM, FCS Orth(SA), MMED(UCT)
Clinical Foot and Ankle Fellow, Chelsea and Westminister Hospital, London,
United Kingdom

ANNE-MARIE O'CONNOR, DBiomechPod, DPodM, MChS, SRCh
Musculo-Skeletal Podiatrist, Fortius Clinic, London, United Kingdom

CHRISTOPHER J. PEARCE, MBChB, FRCS(Orth), MFSEM(UK)
Consultant Orthopaedic Surgeon, Department of Orthopaedics, Alexandra Hospital,
Jurong Healthcare, Singapore, Republic of Singapore

STEFANO PETRILLO, MD
Department of Orthopaedic and Trauma Surgery, Campus Bio-Medico University,
Trigoria; Centro Integrato di Ricerca (CIR), Campus Bio-Medico University, Rome, Italy

WILLIAM JOHN RIBBANS, PhD, FRCSOrth, FFSEM(UK)
Consultant Orthopaedic Surgeon and Professor of Sports Medicine, The University of
Northampton, Northampton, United Kingdom

ANDREW J. ROCHE, MSc, FRCS (Tr & Orth)
Consultant Orthopaedic Surgeon, Chelsea and Westminster Hospital, NHS Foundation
Trust, London, United Kingdom

PETER F. ROSENFELD, FRCS(Tr & Orth)
Consultant Orthopaedic Surgeon, Department of Trauma and Orthopaedics, St Mary's
Hospital, London, United Kingdom

GOWREESON THEVENDRAN, MFSEM (UK), FRCS (Tr & Orth)
Consultant Orthopaedic Surgeon, Department of Orthopaedics, Tan Tock Seng Hospital,
Jalan Tan Tock Seng, Singapore, Republic of Singapore

C. NIEK VAN DIJK, MD, PhD
Department of Orthopedic Surgery, Orthopedic Research Center Amsterdam, Academic
Medical Center, Amsterdam, The Netherlands

ANDY WILLIAMS, FRCS(Orth), FFSEM(UK)
Consultant Orthopaedic Surgeon, Chelsea and Westminster Hospital, London,
United Kingdom

R. LLOYD WILLIAMS, FRCS (Tr & Orth)
Consultant Orthopaedic Surgeon, The London Orthopaedic Clinic, London,
United Kingdom

Contents

Shortest time to union, and to return to sporting activity, are the goals of management of fifth metatarsal fractures in the athlete. Whereas zone 1 injuries are largely treated conservatively, zone 2 and 3 injuries are best treated with surgical fixation in athletes, most commonly with intramedullary screw fixation. Fixation with the addition of bone graft has also yielded good results. In the chronic setting, good results have been shown with intramedullary screw fixation, surgical debridement and bone grafting alone, and tension band wiring. Shock wave therapy and pulsed electromagnetic fields may have a place in chronic and acute injury.

The tibialis posterior tendon and the spring and deltoid ligament complexes combine to provide dynamic and passive stabilization on the medial side of the ankle and hindfoot. Some of the injuries will involve acute injury to previous healthy structures, but many will develop insidiously. The clinician must be aware of new treatment strategies and the level of accompanying scientific evidence regarding injuries sustained by athletes in these areas, while acknowledging that more traditional management applied to nonathletic patients is still likely to be appropriate in the setting of treatment for elite athletes.

Traumatic peroneal tendon subluxation is a rare lesion that occurs most frequently during sporting activities and generally after an ankle sprain. There is consensus regarding the need for surgical stabilization in symptomatic patients, but there is also a general agreement that acute subluxation or dislocations may require surgery in the athlete. Many surgical techniques have been described to treat this lesion. Overall, studies have reported excellent or good results in 90% of cases, although there have been reports of significant complications following open surgical procedures. Endoscopic anatomical retinacular repair offers an attractive alternative to open repair and may reduce complications and allow early return to sports.

The diagnosis of posterior ankle impingement requires an accurate history and specific examination. Computed tomography is a useful investigation to diagnose bony impingement, especially where plain radiography and/or magnetic resonance imaging are sometimes inconclusive. Accurate ultrasound-guided steroid/anesthetic injections are useful interventions to locate the symptomatic lesions and reduce symptoms and occasionally prove curative. If surgical debridement or excision is deemed necessary, arthroscopic surgery via a posterior approach is recommended to excise impingement lesions with a quicker return to sport expected and minimal complications. Open surgical excision, however, remains a viable treatment option.

The incidence of AT rupture has increased in recent decades. AT ruptures frequently occur in the third or fourth decade of life in sedentary individuals who play sport occasionally. Ruptures also occur in elite athletes. Clinical examination must be followed by imaging. Conservative management and early mobilization can achieve excellent results, but the rerupture rate is not acceptable for the management of young, active, or athletic individuals. Open surgery is the most common option for AT ruptures, but there are risks of superficial skin breakdown and wound problems. These problems can be prevented with percutaneous repair.

Tibial diaphyseal stress fractures are rare in the general population, but are more frequently seen in the athletic and military communities. The diagnosis of this problem may be problematic and needs to be considered in all athletes and military recruits who present with shin or ankle pain. The female triad in athletes (low-energy availability/disordered eating, amenorrhea, and osteoporosis/osteopenia) should be considered in those women who sustain this injury. Management is usually conservative with a variety of rehabilitation programs suggested, but a pragmatic approach is to manage the patient symptomatically.

Rehabilitation is easy to do badly and difficult to do well. Many people are involved in the process, and must act as a team to support the patient with good communication and teamwork. The whole process can be satisfying to all concerned when dealing with motivated and enthusiastic patients. Measuring the process is achievable and gives credibility and support to the initial hypothesis of the individual's rehabilitation program. Rehabilitation involves creativity using science and art, with the end result being the patient's return to a normal life or ability to excel within their sport.

Reducing external injury risk factors associated with the boot-surface interaction is important in reducing the incidence and severity of foot and ankle injury. A review of prospective football (soccer) injury epidemiology studies determined that the incidence of noncontact ankle sprain injury is relatively high. Research on the impact of cleat shape and configuration and boot design on the boot-surface interaction is providing new understanding of the impact on player biomechanics and injury risk but is not keeping pace with commercial advances in boot design and innovation in natural and synthetic turf surface technology.

FOOT AND ANKLE CLINICS

DOWNLOAD
Free App!

Review Articles
THE CLINICS

NOW AVAILABLE FOR YOUR iPhone and iPad

Preface

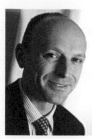

James D.F. Calder, TD, MD, FRCS(Tr & Orth), FFSEM(UK)
Editor

Professional athletes may suffer the same injuries as the rest of us mere mortals but the approach taken to ensure that they return to full fitness in a timely manner may be very different. For some injuries, earlier surgical intervention may enable the strength and conditioning staff to maintain overall fitness during the healing process, while for others, specific rehabilitation techniques may safely shave weeks from their return to a sport program, allowing the player to participate in that "crunch" end-of-season match.

Mark Myerson kindly invited me to put together a group of leading experts who have written informative, sometimes controversial, expert opinion on the optimal management of some of the more common or challenging sporting injuries. There are also 2 articles on subjects that are rarely touched on by orthopedic surgeons (perhaps because of our limited knowledge of their importance). One article gives an overview of the goals and markers used in rehabilitation of the athlete—these may be employed without guidance from the surgeon for major national teams but an understanding of the principles is crucial when developing protocols with second-tier or high-level amateur athletes and their coaching/rehabilitation staff. The second article discusses the influence of the ground-boot interface, the mechanisms of injuries sustained on various playing surfaces, and the basis for recommending specific boots and cleats depending on certain types of foot.

I would like to thank all the authors for their contribution to this issue of *Foot and Ankle Clinics of North America*. Their articles have required minimal editing, making my job as guest editor so much easier! Mark Myerson, a good friend to so many of us, deserves full credit for his tireless dedication as consulting editor of *Foot and*

Foot Ankle Clin N Am 18 (2013) xiii–xiv
http://dx.doi.org/10.1016/j.fcl.2013.02.013
1083-7515/13/$ – see front matter © 2013 Published by Elsevier Inc.

foot.theclinics.com

Ankle Clinics of North America and also as mentor to hundreds of orthopedic surgeons across the globe. I hope that this issue will prove educational and also stimulate further debate.

James D.F. Calder, TD, MD, FRCS(Tr & Orth), FFSEM(UK)
Chelsea & Westminster Hospital
369 Fulham Road
London SW10 9NH, United Kingdom

The Fortius Clinic
17 Fitzhardinge Street
London W1H 6EQ, United Kingdom

E-mail address:
james.calder@imperial.ac.uk

The Role of Ankle Arthroscopy in Acute Ankle Injuries of the Athlete

Steve Hepple, MBChB, FRCS(Tr & Orth)*, Abhijit Guha, FRCS(Tr & Orth)

KEYWORDS

• Athlete • Arthroscopy • Ankle • Sports injury

KEY POINTS

- Up to 60% of ankle fractures may have a cartilage injury.
- Arthroscopy may be helpful in diagnosing intra-articular disease and assessing syndesmosis stability.
- Arthroscopy may assist in the accurate reduction of displaced tibial plafond fractures.

INTRODUCTION

The role of ankle arthroscopy in the management of chronic ankle disease is firmly established, but its use in the acute setting is less well defined and the range of indications for such arthroscopic or arthroscopically assisted procedures have not been clearly identified. Various investigators advocate its use in a wide variety of situations, but the evidence for use in such cases is generally restricted to level 4 evidence (**Box 1**). The potential benefits of performing minimal access or arthroscopic surgery are clear in the athlete with potential for accelerated rehabilitation and return to sport. Consequently, there is growing appreciation that acute arthroscopic assessment or arthroscopic-assisted treatment of acute injuries cannot only match the outcomes of traditional open surgery but in many situations considerably enhances our techniques and therefore has a key role to play in the setting of acute ankle injury of the athlete. It is likely that the spectrum of disease amenable to arthroscopic treatment will expand over the next decade and further more powerful evidence for this should be a priority.

ACUTE ANKLE LIGAMENT INJURY

Acute ankle sprain injury is the most common acute sport trauma, accounting for about 14% of all sport-related injuries.[1] Most ankle sprain injuries are believed to be

Disclosures: None.
Department of Orthopaedics, Avon Orthopaedic Centre, Southmead Hospital, Southmead Road, Bristol BS10 5NB, UK
* Corresponding author.
E-mail address: steve.hepple@nbt.nhs.uk

Foot Ankle Clin N Am 18 (2013) 185–194
http://dx.doi.org/10.1016/j.fcl.2013.02.001
1083-7515/13/$ – see front matter © 2013 Elsevier Inc. All rights reserved.

Box 1
Indications for acute ankle arthroscopy

Indications for arthroscopic-assisted surgery in acute ankle injuries

- Acute ligament injury
- Chondral/osteochondral injuries
- Malleolar fracture
- Distal tibial fracture
- Syndesmotic injuries
- Talus body/neck fractures
- Talar process fractures
- Periankle tendoscopy

caused by incorrect foot positioning at the point of landing. The ground reaction force is deviated medially and this causes a sudden supination or inversion moment at the subtalar joint. Another proposed cause is the delayed reaction time of the peroneal muscles at the lateral aspect of the ankle.[1]

Surgical intervention in acute ligament injuries remains controversial. The Cochrane database review[2] concluded that there was no benefit of acute surgical intervention versus conservative treatment, but many of the included studies were methodologically flawed, making interpretation difficult. More recent individual randomized studies suggest lower rates of pain and recurrent instability in the surgical group, but the differences are subtle.[3]

There is little doubt that most low-to-moderate-demand individuals suffering an isolated lateral ligament injury should be treated conservatively with the expectation that a full recovery to normal sporting function will occur after appropriate functional rehabilitation. Failing this recovery and in the presence of ongoing symptoms of instability, a late anatomic repair/reconstruction of the lateral ligaments has been shown to produce excellent results at least equivalent to the results achieved by acute repair.

Most investigators therefore consider acute surgical repair of the lateral ligaments only in the high-demand patient or athlete to enhance and accelerate the return to normal training and activity.

In these situations, simultaneous acute arthroscopic assessment of the joint is considered appropriate. It is now well documented that intra-articular joint surface damage is common in the sprained ankle. Much of this damage is confined to the chondral surface and does not involve underlying bone. In these circumstances, magnetic resonance imaging (MRI) does not always show the lesion. Komenda and Ferkel[4] reported an incidence of up to 93% of intra-articular disease in patients undergoing arthroscopy immediately before lateral ligament repair, whereas others have shown as little as 40% sensitivity of MRI to coexistent intra-articular lesions after lateral ligament injury.[5,6] Although most of these studies relate to the chronic situation, it is reasonable to assume that a percentage of acutely diagnosed lateral ligament injuries undergoing early surgery have combined intra-articular disease either not visible on MRI or obscured by acute edema/hemorrhage.

It is clear, therefore, that acute ankle arthroscopy in these cases has potentially significant benefits in detecting lesions that may prevent or hamper recovery after an otherwise successful ligament repair.

Although some surgeons prefer not to combine an arthroscopic procedure with ligament repair because of the effects of fluid extravasation into the soft tissues, this is rarely a clinical issue, and the benefit of being able to fully examine the joint before it is stabilized by the ligament repair outweighs any negative effects of fluid leaking into the soft tissues. Staging the procedures seems unnecessary.

There is no evidence to guide surgeons encountering these lesions in the acute phase as to which lesions are those that cause late ongoing symptoms and hence should be treated versus those that would settle spontaneously if left undetected. Some such lesions may therefore be overtreated, and more work is required to clarify the issue.

Recently, some investigators have described novel techniques to achieve lateral ligament stabilization by entirely arthroscopic means. These techniques remain experimental and have been reported only in cases of chronic instability. With improving techniques, this indication may be expanded to acute management.[7,8]

CHONDRAL/OSTEOCHONDRAL LESIONS

Injuries to the articular surface of the ankle are common after ankle trauma and are one of the most frequent causes of failure to settle after acute ankle injury. They can occur both after apparent simple sprains or in combination with other ankle fractures. Ferkel[9] showed that up to 60% of ankle fractures undergoing surgical fixation demonstrated evidence of articular surface damage, most of which were undiagnosed before surgery because of the low sensitivity of plain radiography (often the only imaging modality used in an acute isolated malleolar fracture).

Although much has been published regarding the management of osteochondral lesions of the talus, most of this material relates to the chronic situation. The natural history of purely chondral surface damage is not established. The findings of Ferkel suggest that many such lesions go undiagnosed and apparently settle down without long-term symptoms after rehabilitation from the more major injury. The active treatment of some of these lesions in the acute setting is therefore open to question, and further high-level evidence is required.

Although only a small percentage of osteochondral lesions are diagnosed early, they are often those most amenable to early arthroscopic treatment, because they tend to be displaced lesions with a substantial bony component easily visible on plain radiographs. In the case of an acute presentation of an obviously displaced osteochondral lesion, then early arthroscopic assessment is clearly indicated. Direct arthroscopic visualization of the lesion allows assessment of the site, size, and condition of the fragment. The presence of a substantial bony element and the condition of the donor site determine whether an acute fixation or fragment removal is performed.

When appropriate, these lesions can and should be reimplanted either entirely arthroscopically or through a small arthrotomy with arthroscopic assistance. Stable fixation is achieved with either headless screws or bioabsorbable pins. This fixation is best performed in the acute setting before subtle bony swelling and deformity caused by persistent weight bearing alter the anatomic fit of the fragment.

If deemed nonsalvageable, then any loose fragments may be excised and the surrounding edges of the lesion stabilized via arthroscopic means. Subsequently, the bed of the donor site should be treated by some marrow stimulation technique such as drilling, abrasion, or microfracture. This treatment stimulates in-growth of a fibrocartilaginous plug, and current evidence suggests that in lesions up to 150 mm^2, this produces good medium-term to long-term results in 80% or more of patients.[10,11] In most cases, this result can be achieved by routine 2-portal anterior arthroscopic techniques, but occasionally, a supplementary anterior portal or posterior portal is required to complete the procedure.

In cases in which the initial lesion is assessed at 150 mm^2 or greater and immediate fixation of an osteochondral fragment is not possible, there is substantial evidence to suggest that marrow stimulation techniques have a poorer outcome than in the smaller lesions.[10,11] Early second-line intervention in this scenario is being popularized. Techniques such as autologous chondrocyte implantation, matrix-assisted autologous chondrocyte inplantation (MACI), mosaicoplasty, bulk allografting, local stem cell or platelet-rich plasma therapy with or without bioactive membrane implantation, bone substitute plugs, or metallic resurfacing have all been proposed. The initial early arthroscopy can therefore be used to assess the size of the lesion precisely, and in the case of cartilage growth techniques, a suitable biopsy from the edge of the lesion can be taken and stored in the laboratory. If the initial debridement fails to settle the symptoms, then the cells may be cultured and used for reimplantation at a later date. Arthroscopic reimplantation by MACI is now a technical reality.[12]

There is no consensus amongst foot and ankle surgeons on the most appropriate second-line treatment. Most patients undergoing these treatment strategies should therefore be the subject of rigorous follow-up and ideally entered into further prospective trials.

In contrast to lesions affecting the talus, there is little published evidence regarding osteochondral defects of the tibial plafond. They present considerably less frequently (approximately 7% of all ankle osteochondral injuries[13]), and the trend is to treat along the same principles as talus lesions. The results of a few small series suggest that the medium-term outcome after simple acute debridement and marrow stimulation is equal to or slightly inferior to the results in treatment of talus lesions.[14]

SYNDESMOTIC INJURY

Some degree of syndesmotic ligament injury is reported to occur in 47% to 66% of Weber B and C ankle fractures.[9,15] Diagnosis is often difficult, particularly when plain radiography is relied on. Stress radiography increases the sensitivity of diagnosis, as does computed tomography (CT) or MRI scanning[16–18]; however, no radiographic technique is entirely reliable, and abnormal values of many radiographic indices used vary between investigators, making the assessment of syndesmotic injury controversial. Syndesmotic instability can also occur without any bony trauma (the so-called high ankle sprain), and in such cases, a high index of diagnostic suspicion is required.

There is increasing evidence that arthroscopic assessment of the syndesmosis has greater accuracy than static or stressed radiological assessment.[15,19,20] At arthroscopy, easy passage of the arthroscope into the lateral gutter is suspicious for instability, and further information is gained by unhindered passage of instruments into the tibiofibular recess (Fig. 1). Torn anterior and posterior inferior tibiofibular ligaments can be directly visualized, although the interosseous ligament is less visible. External stress placed on the fibula allows observation of the stability in various planes. Damage to the medial ridge of the talus is commonly associated with syndesmotic injury.[21]

Untreated, syndesmotic instability can undoubtedly result in persistent long-term symptoms in the ankle, and therefore improved diagnostic accuracy is potentially of great benefit. Burns and colleagues[22] showed that complete disruption of the syndesmosis produces 40% reduction in contact surface area. Advocates of the arthroscopic technique to diagnose syndesmotic injuries suggest that the increased diagnosis of traumatic instability may be caused by the ability of direct visualization to detect instability in more than the coronal plane. Plain radiographic techniques and published indices

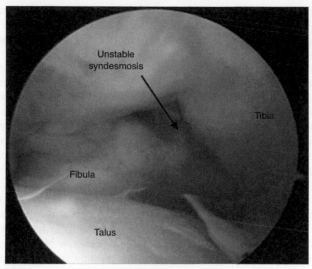

Fig. 1. Unstable syndesmosis viewed arthroscopically.

for the assessment of the syndesmosis make no reference to the possibility of instability in the sagittal, longitudinal, or rotational planes, which are more easily visualized at arthroscopy. A revised classification scheme has been proposed taking into account all planes of possible instability and distinguishing between frank (diagnosed on radiographs) and occult (diagnosed only by arthroscopy) instability (**Table 1**).[15]

Although the evidence points to an underdiagnosis of syndesmotic instability with traditional methods, it is not clear how the syndesmosis should be managed after arthroscopically assisted diagnosis. The use of this technique may lead to overtreatment of the problem, and further work is required to establish at what level of arthroscopically diagnosed instability intervention is required, although in the athlete, current opinion indicates an aggressive debridement and stabilization approach.

Ogilvie-Harris and Reed[23] reported good results in 19 patients after simple debridement of the unstable syndesmosis after ankle fracture, but other investigators have chosen, in addition, to stabilize the syndesmosis by percutaneous fixation; in similar-sized series by Wolf and Amendola[24] and Liu and colleagues,[15] good outcomes were observed.

MALLEOLAR FRACTURE

Malleolar fractures of all types requiring reduction and internal fixation are universally managed by open or minimal access approaches, but ankle arthroscopy can be

Table 1		
Syndesmosis diastasis classification		
A Frank		**B Occult**
1 Coronal	Can be detected by arthroscopy or stress radiographs	1 Coronal
2 Sagittal	Can be detected by ankle arthroscopy	2 Sagittal
3 Rotational	Can be detected by ankle arthroscopy	3 Rotational
4 Longitudinal	Can be detected by plain radiography	4 Longitudinal

Data from Lui TH, Ip K, Chow HT. Comparison of radiologic and arthroscopic diagnoses of distal tibiofibular syndesmosis disruption in acute ankle fracture. Arthroscopy 2005;21(11):1370.

useful, particularly in cases that are fixed via small incisions. The arthroscope can be used to assist with and ascertain accuracy of anatomic reduction of the fracture and ensure that there is no internal abnormality around the fracture site at the completion of the procedure.

There is a substantial incidence, reported at up to 75%, of coexistent intra-articular damage apart from the fracture site in ankle fractures.[25,26] This damage is most commonly cartilaginous in nature and therefore not radiographically visible. These lesions usually occur at sites not accessible by traditional incisions for fracture surgery, and therefore simultaneous arthroscopic assessment and management of these lesions is required, which should improve the rate and quality of recovery after fracture surgery.

In the only prospective randomized trial comparing arthroscopically assisted with traditional nonassisted lateral malleolar fracture fixation, Takao and colleagues[26] showed a high rate of secondary disease (mostly chondral damage and syndesmotic injury). They reported a small but significantly greater American Orthopaedic Foot and Ankle Society score in the arthroscopically assisted group at average follow-up of 40 months, but the benefit was confined to those fractures classified as pronation abduction types according to the Lauge-Hansen classification. Further work is therefore required to clarify the indications for this intervention.

DISTAL TIBIAL FRACTURE

In the adolescent athlete, the pattern of distal tibial growth plate arrest predisposes this area to unusual intra-articular fracture patterns such as triplane and Tillaux fractures. These fractures in the younger population undoubtedly benefit from arthroscopically assisted reduction and fixation to produce as near anatomic restoration of the joint surface as possible. In the mature athlete, certain partial articular fractures (AO type B3) should also respond well to similar techniques, allowing clearance of the fracture site and accurate realignment. Complete articular assessment for other simultaneous disease can be performed. Often chondral damage is observed on the opposing talar surface, and this is not ordinarily detected preoperatively by either radiographs or CT scanning.

The technique is particularly attractive for the management of simple posterior malleolar fractures, in which direct visualization of the fracture line and reduction can otherwise involve large exposures.

Articular distraction by either skeletal or soft tissue traction is recommended in these cases. Gravity-fed fluid inflow is preferred to pump devices to avoid the risk of secondary calf compartment syndrome. The arthroscopic element of the procedure is used to identify the fracture pattern, clear any comminution or depressed fragments, and aid reduction of the fracture. K-wires may be percutaneously inserted into the fracture fragments to manipulate them into position before definitive fixation is usually achieved via cannulated lag screw techniques. Large plates are not usually required for these fracture patterns.

Results of this technique seem encouraging, with all investigators reporting good outcomes and early return to full activity using the technique in both adolescent and adult fractures; however, the technique is demanding and the published evidence consists only of small groups or single case reports.[27-31] No comparisons are made with conventional open techniques.

TALUS BODY/NECK FRACTURES

Fractures of the talar body and neck are rare injuries, resulting in significant morbidity and complications. In the athletic individual, this type of fracture is highly likely to have a deleterious affect on the long-term functional outcome. The result is determined by the quality of the reduction and preservation of the talus blood supply, and it has been proposed that arthroscopically assisted techniques confer benefit in both of these aspects. Saltzman and colleagues[32] have described their technique but admit that this technique is limited to the simpler 2-part fracture patterns or those that require some debridement of minimal comminution at the fracture site. The technique is demanding and prolongs operative time as well as increasing soft tissue swelling. Case reports or small series[32,33] provide little evidence on which to recommend this technique.

TALAR PROCESS INJURIES

These injuries are usually fractures of the lateral or posterior process and comprise some of the most commonly missed fractures in the acute ankle injury.

Routine anteroposterior and lateral radiographs often do not show the acute fracture, and even specialist views can be incorrectly interpreted. CT scanning remains the mainstay of diagnosis, but before this is performed, a high index of suspicion is required by the assessing physician.

Lateral process fractures occur commonly in snowboarders, who often present with the symptoms and signs of a simple ankle sprain. Undiagnosed and untreated, these fractures can often lead to persistent lateral ankle pain and late subtalar joint arthritis. Outcomes are poorer when diagnosis and treatment are delayed more than 2 weeks.[34] The classification of these fractures is shown in **Box 2**.

Type 1 fractures benefit from stable fixation, usually via an open surgical technique. Type 3 fractures respond well to conservative treatment. However, type 2 fractures seem to respond best to early removal of the fracture fragments rather than delayed surgery. Removal of these fracture fragments by arthroscopic means reduces the surrounding soft tissue dissection and potentially accelerates return to normal activity, although there are no published results regarding this technique.

Posterior process fractures occur usually as a result of forced plantar flexion injuries and are even less common than lateral process fractures. Most of these injuries are treated initially with conservative treatment, but in the athletic population, a few cases with significant comminution may be appropriately treated by early arthroscopic debridement.

PERONEAL TENDON INJURIES

Peroneal tendon tears were first described by Meyer in 1924,[35] initially as an attritional disease, but current theory suggests that they are mainly mechanical, occurring after a traumatic episode, rather than degenerative in nature. In the athlete presenting with

---

Box 2
Hawkins classification of lateral talar process fractures

Lateral talar process fractures

Type 1: simple fracture extending from talofibular to talocalcaneal joint

Type 2: commminuted fracture

Type 3: small chip fracture not involving talofibular joint

Data from Hawkins LG. Fracture of the lateral process of the talus. J Bone Joint Surg Am 1965;47(6):1170–5.

acute ankle injury, the diagnosis of peroneal tendon injury needs to be carefully considered to avoid late presentation. Various intrinsic and extrinsic factors have been implicated in peroneal tendon tears.[36] Intrinsic factors include a flat fibular groove, a low-lying muscle belly, osteophytic spurring, laxity of superior peroneal retinaculum, and a cavus foot. Extrinsic factors mainly involve the sporting activity and foot position on impact.

They are commonly misdiagnosed as ankle sprains and are often associated with lateral ankle instability or intra-articular disease. Bare and Ferkel[36] reported 60 intra-articular lesions in 30 ankles undergoing peroneal tendon repair, with each patient having between 1 and 3 lesions. The ankle disease included soft tissue impingement, loose bodies, osteochondral lesions, extensive scar tissue, extensive synovitis, and anterior osteophytes. Most (78%) of these lesions were undetected on preoperative scans. These investigators proposed that ankle arthroscopy should be routinely performed while undertaking peroneal tendon repair, and this is certainly indicated in the acute athletic setting.

Endoscopy of the peroneal sheath is gaining popularity in the management of peroneal tendon dysfunction.[37] The published literature contains only reports of this technique as a treatment tool performed in the chronic situation, and the therapeutic techniques that are technically possible are limited mainly to simple debridement in the sheath. However, in the acute setting, tendoscopy can in certain situations be a useful diagnostic tool and can accurately localize the site of injury, allowing repair through a limited incision.

Ankle arthroscopy should therefore be routinely undertaken in the presence of an acute peroneal tendon tear. This strategy enables early detection and treatment of intra-articular lesions invisible to imaging techniques. Further work is required to develop the therapeutic rather than purely diagnostic benefits of peroneal tendoscopy in the acute setting.

REFERENCES

1. Fong DT, Chan YY, Mok KM, et al. Understanding acute ankle ligamentous strain injury in sports. Sports Med Arthrosc Rehabil Ther Technol 2009;1–14.
2. Kerkhoffs GM, Handoll HH, de Bie R, et al. Surgical versus conservative treatment for acute injuries of the lateral ligament complex of the ankle in adults [review]. Cochrane Database Syst Rev 2007;(2):CD000380.
3. Pijnenburg AC, Bogaard K, Krips R, et al. Operative and functional treatment of rupture of the lateral ligament of the ankle. A randomised, prospective trial. J Bone Joint Surg Br 2003;85(4):525–30.
4. Kemonda GA, Ferkel RD. Arthroscopic findings associated with the unstable ankle. Foot Ankle Int 1999;20:708–13.
5. Joshy S, Abdulkadir U, Chaganti S, et al. Accuracy of MRI scan in the diagnosis of ligamentous and chondral pathology in the ankle. Foot Ankle Surg 2010;16(2):78–80.
6. O'Neill PJ, Van Aman SE, Guyton GP. Is MRI adequate to detect lesions in patients with ankle instability? Clin Orthop Relat Res 2010;468(4):1115–9.
7. Lui TH. Arthroscopy and endoscopy of the foot and ankle: indications for new techniques [review]. Arthroscopy 2007;23(8):889–902.
8. Corte-Real NM, Moreira RM. Arthroscopic repair of chronic lateral ankle instability. Foot Ankle Int 2009;30(3):213–7.
9. Loren GJ, Ferkel RD. Arthroscopic assessment of occult intra-articular injury in acute ankle fractures. Arthroscopy 2002;18(4):412–21.

10. Cuttica DJ, Smith WB, Hyer CF, et al. Osteochondral lesions of the talus: predictors of clinical outcome. Foot Ankle Int 2011;32(11):1045–51.
11. Choi WJ, Park KK, Kim BS, et al. Osteochondral lesion of the talus: is there a critical defect size for poor outcome? Am J Sports Med 2009;37(10):1974–80.
12. Aurich M, Bedi HS, Smith PJ, et al. Arthroscopic treatment of osteochondral lesions of the ankle with matrix-associated chondrocyte implantation: early clinical and magnetic resonance imaging results. Am J Sports Med 2011;39(2):311–9.
13. Elias I, Raikin SM, Schweitzer ME, et al. Osteochondral lesions of the distal tibial plafond: localization and morphologic characteristics with an anatomical grid. Foot Ankle Int 2009;30(6):524–9.
14. Mologne TS, Ferkel RD. Arthroscopic treatment of osteochondral lesions of the distal tibia. Foot Ankle Int 2007;28(8):865–72.
15. Lui TH, Ip K, Chow HT. Comparison of radiologic and arthroscopic diagnoses of distal tibiofibular syndesmosis disruption in acute ankle fracture. Arthroscopy 2005;21(11):1370.
16. Gardner MJ, Demetrakopoulos D, Briggs SM, et al. Malreduction of the tibiofibular syndesmosis in ankle fractures. Foot Ankle Int 2006;27(10):788–92.
17. Oae K, Takao M, Naito K, et al. Injury of the tibiofibular syndesmosis: value of MR imaging for diagnosis. Radiology 2003;227(1):155–61.
18. Vogl TJ, Hochmuth K, Diebold T, et al. Magnetic resonance imaging in the diagnosis of acute injured distal tibiofibular syndesmosis. Invest Radiol 1997;32(7):401–9.
19. Takao M, Ochi M, Naito K, et al. Arthroscopic diagnosis of tibiofibular syndesmosis disruption. Arthroscopy 2001;17(8):836–43.
20. Sri-Ram K, Robinson AH. Arthroscopic assessment of the syndesmosis following ankle fracture. Injury 2005;36(5):675–8.
21. Yoshimura I, Naito M, Kanazawa K, et al. Arthroscopic findings in Maisonneuve fractures. J Orthop Sci 2008;13(1):3–6.
22. Burns WC 2nd, Prakash K, Adelaar R, et al. Tibiotalar joint dynamics: indications for the syndesmotic screw–a cadaver study. Foot Ankle 1993;14(3):153–8.
23. Ogilvie-Harris DJ, Reed SC. Disruption of the ankle syndesmosis: diagnosis and treatment by arthroscopic surgery. Arthroscopy 1994;10(5):561–8.
24. Wolf BR, Amendola A. Syndesmosis injuries in the athlete: when and how to operate. Curr Opin Orthop 2002;13:151–4.
25. Ono A, Nishikawa S, Nagao A, et al. Arthroscopically assisted treatment of ankle fractures: arthroscopic findings and surgical outcomes. Arthroscopy 2004;20(6):627–31.
26. Takao M, Uchio Y, Naito K, et al. Diagnosis and treatment of combined intra-articular disorders in acute distal fibular fractures. J Trauma 2004;57(6):1303–7.
27. McGillion S, Jackson M, Lahoti O. Arthroscopically assisted percutaneous fixation of triplane fracture of the distal tibia. J Pediatr Orthop B 2007;16(5):313–6.
28. Panagopoulos A, van Niekerk L. Arthroscopic assisted reduction and fixation of a juvenile Tillaux fracture. Knee Surg Sports Traumatol Arthrosc 2007;15(4):415–7.
29. Imade S, Takao M, Nishi H, et al. Arthroscopy-assisted reduction and percutaneous fixation for triplane fracture of the distal tibia. Arthroscopy 2004;20(10):e123–8.
30. Whipple TL, Martin DR, McIntyre LF, et al. Arthroscopic treatment of triplane fractures of the ankle. Arthroscopy 1993;9(4):456–63.
31. Cetik O, Cift H, Ari M, et al. Arthroscopy-assisted combined external and internal fixation of a pilon fracture of the tibia. Hong Kong Med J 2007;13(5):403–5.

32. Saltzman CL, Marsh JL, Tearse DS. Treatment of displaced talus fractures: an arthroscopically assisted approach. Foot Ankle Int 1994;15(11):630–3.
33. Subairy A, Subramanian K, Geary NP. Arthroscopically assisted internal fixation of a talus body fracture [Erratum appears in Injury 2004;35(1):104]. Injury 2004;35(1): 86–9.
34. Perera A, Baker JF, Lui DF, et al. The management and outcome of lateral process fracture of the talus [review]. Foot Ankle Surg 2010;16(1):15–20.
35. Meyer AW. Further evidence of attrition in the human body. Am J Anat 1924;34: 241–61.
36. Bare A, Ferkel RD. Peroneal tendon tears: associated arthroscopic findings and results after repair. Arthroscopy 2009;25(11):1288–97.
37. Sammarco VJ. Peroneal tendoscopy: indications and techniques. Sports Med Arthrosc 2009;17:94–9.

Management of Syndesmosis Injuries in the Elite Athlete

May Fong Mak, MBChB, MRCS, MMed Ortho[a],
Louise Gartner, MBBS, MRCP, FRCR[b],
Christopher J. Pearce, MBChB, FRCS(Orth), MFSEM(UK)[c,*]

KEYWORDS

• Syndesmosis • Tibiofibular • Injury • Athlete • Elite • Treatment • Controversies

KEY POINTS

• Late diagnosis of unstable syndesmosis injuries leads to a poor outcome and delayed return to sports.
• A high index of suspicion is required with understanding of the mechanism of injury to ensure an early diagnosis.
• Incomplete and/or inaccurate reduction leads to a poor outcome.

INTRODUCTION

A syndesmosis injury or "high ankle sprain" is a significant injury, especially in the elite athlete. It constitutes a spectrum of injury, ranging from a simple ligamentous sprain to frank diastasis with concomitant bone, osteochondral, and/or soft-tissue injury. It has been shown to be associated with a longer recovery period and greater functional impairment compared with any other type of ankle sprain.[1–6] Of all ankle sprains, the syndesmotic injury is most predictive of persistent symptoms in the athletic population.[7]

Sprains of the syndesmosis without frank diastasis or fracture are the commonest variety seen in athletes. Estimates on the incidence of syndesmosis injuries are reported to vary broadly, from 1% to 18% of all ankle sprains.[8] The differences in reporting may in part be attributable to a lack of clear diagnostic criteria and a low index of suspicion for this injury, with mild sprains commonly being underdiagnosed or misdiagnosed. Undertreatment of these injuries can lead to significant morbidity, as instability and posttraumatic arthritis may ensue.[9–12]

The authors have nothing to disclose.
[a] Department of Orthopaedics, Khoo Teck Puat Hospital, 90 Yishun Central, Singapore 768828, Republic of Singapore; [b] Department of Radiology, National University Hospital, 21 Lower Kent Ridge Road, Singapore 119077, Republic of Singapore; [c] Department of Orthopaedics, Alexandra Hospital, Jurong Healthcare, 378 Alexandra Road, Singapore 159964, Republic of Singapore
* Corresponding author.
E-mail address: chris.pearce@doctors.net.uk

Foot Ankle Clin N Am 18 (2013) 195–214
http://dx.doi.org/10.1016/j.fcl.2013.02.002
1083-7515/13/$ – see front matter © 2013 Elsevier Inc. All rights reserved.

Normal biomechanics of the ankle syndesmosis is essential for weight bearing, with reports pertaining to this in the literature dating back to 1773, by Bromfield.[13] More than a century later, Quenu[14] published on tibiofibular diastasis as a result of ligamentous disruption. The recognition of this injury generated further research and has raised many of the controversial topics that we face today. Our ability to clinically diagnose, image, classify injury severity, stratify treatment, and predict a safe return to high-level sport has improved, but many aspects of this topic remain enigmatic.

This article reviews the basics and evidence base thus far on syndesmosis injuries, with a focus on its management in the elite sporting population.

ANATOMY

The ligamentous connection between the tibia and fibula may be anatomically defined to consist of the proximal tibiofibular syndesmosis, the interosseous membrane (IOM), and the distal tibiofibular syndesmotic complex. The distal syndesmosis complex may be further divided into its 5 components[8] as follows.

The anterior inferior tibiofibular ligament (AITFL) is an anterior structure that traverses the joint at an oblique 45° angle from the anterior tubercle (Chaput tubercle) of the tibia to the anterior aspect of the distal fibula (Wagstaffe tubercle). It is often multifascicular with 2 or 3 parallel portions. It is approximately 16 mm in length, and averages 16 and 13 mm wide at its tibial origin and fibular insertion, respectively.[15] The AITFL is the commonest part of the distal syndesmotic complex to be torn.[16]

The posterior inferior tibiofibular ligament (PITFL) is the strongest portion of the complex and lies in the posterior part of the syndesmosis. From its origin at the posterior tubercle of the tibia, it descends posterolaterally to insert into the posterior aspect of the distal fibula. On average, its length is 20 mm and its width measurements are 18 and 12 mm at its tibial origin and fibular insertion, respectively. Compared with the AITFL, the superiority of the strength and load to failure of the PITFL renders it the syndesmotic structure least likely to be injured during trauma.[17,18]

The transverse tibiofibular ligament (TTFL) has a fibrocartilagenous appearance that functions akin to a labrum. It deepens the tibiotalar articulation and reinforces the posterior capsule of the ankle joint. It is frequently referred to as the deep portion of the PITFL. The ligament originates from the medial part of the tibia and runs horizontally until it inserts on the posterior tubercle of the fibula.

The pyramid-shaped interosseous ligament (IOL) has strong and short fanlike fibers that occupy the distal tibiofibular space.[19] The IOL forms the main attachment between the tibia and fibula. It is positioned 0.5 to 2.0 cm above the joint line and within the pivot of the rotational plane of the distal fibula.[20,21]

The distal portion of the IOM is a direct continuation of the IOL. The IOM connects the tibia and fibula throughout their lengths, and plays only a minimal role as a stabilizer of the syndesmosis.[22]

The inherent stability of the distal tibiofibular joint is also contributed to by the bony articulation formed through the containment of the distal fibula in the incisura fibularis of the distal tibia. The morphology of the incisura fibularis depends on the size of the tibial tubercles that form the anterior and posterior margins of the groove. The most common variety seen in a cadaveric study was concave (75%), followed by convex (16%), with the small remainder described as irregular and therefore could not be grouped as a specific pattern.[21] In another cadaveric study, the depth of concavity within the concave group was shown to differ between being significantly concave (60%) to "shallowly concave" (40%).[23] A study based on computed tomography (CT) imaging of 100 normal distal tibiofibular syndesmoses showed variation of the articulation between genders, with variation between the anterior and posterior dimensions within the syndesmosis.[24] Evidently the great diversity of the articulation poses both diagnostic and operative challenges to the practitioner; the radiographic evaluation of diastasis becomes unclear, and attempts to obtain anatomic reduction of the joint may be technically difficult in the nonconcave group.

BIOMECHANICS

The talus is broad anteriorly and laterally, and has an axis that lies obliquely. This irregular shape renders the ankle joint more complex than a simple hinge joint, as the distal fibula is thought to rotate externally, and translate proximally and laterally during normal ankle dorsiflexion to accommodate the irregularly shaped talus.[25] The width of the ankle joint is thus dynamic during physiologic motion while the distal tibiofibular articulation is held stable by the strong confluence of syndesmotic ligaments.

In the static stance phase, the ankle joint is stable and suited well to bear pressures that are equal to the individual's body weight.[8] By contrast, a multitude of different forces passes through the foot and ankle during vigorous athletic activity. This region sustains enormous stress that may disrupt the mortise during high-level sports injury. Syndesmotic ligament rupture usually occurs as a result of a significant external rotation force. Ogilvie-Harris and Reed[26] found that the AITFL contributed 35%, the TTFL 33%, the IOL 22%, and the PITFL 9% to the overall tibiofibular stability when these ligaments were serially cut in a cadaveric study. The investigators concluded that disruption to 2 of the ligaments would compromise the resistance of the syndesmosis by half and cause instability. In another sectioning study, Xenos and colleagues[27] demonstrated progressive increase in diastasis with sequential sectioning of the ligaments in the cadaveric syndesmosis. Talus translation of 2.3 mm after complete transection of the AITFL increased to a talar translation of 7.3 mm with external rotation, averaging 10.2° when all of the ligaments were sectioned.

Abnormal pressures at the ankle joint can result from seemingly minor disruptions of the mortise. The distal fibula that is translated laterally 1 to 2 mm, shortened 2 mm, and externally rotated 5° will significantly decrease the contact area between the tibia and talus through deformation of the mortise, and these parameters are enough to be precursors to end-stage ankle arthritis stemming from pathologic joint-pressure redistribution.[28–30] In their classic article, Ramsey and Hamilton[28] demonstrated that stress per unit area increased as the total tibiotalar contact area decreased. One millimeter of lateral displacement of the talus represented a 42% reduction in contact area between the talus and tibia. The cadaveric biomechanical study on the effect of fibular displacement in a pronation–lateral rotation ankle fracture malunion model by Thordarson and colleagues[30] showed that any measure of shortening, external rotation, or lateral translation, alone or in combination, led to decreased contact area and hence increased contact pressures.

MECHANISM OF INJURY

The commonest described mechanism of syndesmotic injury involves an external rotation moment at the ankle with the foot positioned in dorsiflexion and pronation.[27] The talus in the ankle mortise is forcibly externally rotated against the fibula, thus separating the fibula from the tibia; this tensions and ruptures the AITFL first. As external rotation continues, disruption of the IOL and IOM follows, and finally rupture or avulsion of the PITFL and TTFL occurs. The fibula may fracture in the final stage of this injury with persistently applied force. In addition to injuring the syndesmotic ligaments, the initial external rotation of the talus on the tibia may also disrupt the medial deltoid ligament or instead may cause a medial malleolar fracture. Isolated complete ruptures and diastasis of the syndesmosis were traditionally considered rare,[31] and most of the injuries were reported to be associated with malleolar or proximal fibular (Maisonneuve) fractures. However, with increasing sports participation around the world as well as a greater awareness of the injury and more sophisticated imaging, clinicians will see ever more of these injuries in practice.

Athletes who participate in sports such as American football, hockey, rugby, wrestling, and lacrosse are at higher risk of sustaining syndesmotic injuries.[1,3,32,33] These sports demand twisting and cutting actions, and a great level of intensity. In collision sports such as American football, the talus is violently external-rotated when a force is applied to the proximal leg or body of an athlete whose foot is planted firmly on the ground; for example, during a tackle or when a downward force is applied to an athlete in prone position whose foot is held in external rotation, commonly in a pile-up. In slalom skiing and hockey, the use of boots to immobilize the athlete's ankle, and hence protect the ankle ligaments (AITFL, calcaneofibular ligament, and deltoid ligament), makes the syndesmosis susceptible to injury when an external rotation force is applied. In skiing, this typically occurs when the skier's ski tip gets caught in the gate when the skier is moving at high speed. In rodeo, the downed rider sustains the injury when the bull tramples on the lateral side of the rider's ankle. These sports are not unique in predisposing the elite athlete to syndesmosis injuries, ranging from sprains to latent or frank diastases and fractures. Syndesmosis injuries in this population account for 75% of all ankle injuries, compared with a considerably lower rate of 10% to 20% of all ankle sprains in the general athletic population,[7,34] and a rate of 1% to 17% of all ankle injuries in the normal population.[3,7,32]

CLINICAL EVALUATION

A methodical history to determine the mechanism of injury and a thorough physical examination are crucial to making the diagnosis of a syndesmotic injury. The symptoms of pain, swelling, and difficulty with ambulation are general to most ankle trauma, and the self-reported history about the "ankle sprain" sustained during high-impact or high-speed sports is frequently unclear. Hence, the practitioner needs to maintain a high index of suspicion to glean relevant and precise details regarding the mechanism of injury, the first guiding clue toward differentiating a syndesmotic injury from other lateral ankle injuries. It is also imperative to document the interval between injury and clinical presentation. The temporal classification of acute (<3 weeks), subacute (3 weeks to 3 months), or chronic (>3 months) will have a bearing on the management of these injuries.[22]

As in all ankle injuries, the physical examination of the ankle must involve a systematic approach. The examination should begin with an appreciation of ecchymosis and soft-tissue edema in the anterolateral aspect of the ankle. The classic physical examination finding in patients with acute syndesmosis injuries is well-localized tenderness in the anterior space between tibia and fibula. The distance this tenderness extends proximally, coined the tenderness length, has a strong correlation with the degree of injury and time of return to sports activity.[32] Palpation of the malleoli and other bony landmarks including the proximal fibula, as well as major ligamentous areas must be included to assess for associated problems.

Several provocative tests for the evaluation of syndesmosis injuries have been described, with the squeeze test and the external rotation test being the most commonly cited. These special tests use the reproducibility of pain to increase the accuracy of a clinical diagnosis of syndesmosis injury. However, their ability to accurately or consistently diagnose, prognosticate, or stratify the severity of mechanical instability remains uncertain.[35] In the squeeze test (**Fig. 1**), pain is replicated at the level of the ankle joint as the distal tibia and fibula separate when the leg is compressed at or slightly above mid-calf level. In the external rotation test (**Fig. 2**), the ankle is dorsiflexed and the foot is externally rotated to replicate the mechanism of injury, and pain indicates a positive test. The external rotation test may also be achieved with the patient standing and rotating his or her body with the foot planted on the floor. In addition, the fibula translation test, Cotton test, and crossed-leg test also have roles in diagnosis of syndesmosis injuries.[36,37] When performing the fibular translation test, the examiner attempts to move the fibula in the anterior-posterior plane; increased translation and pain in comparison with the other ankle suggests an injury to the syndesmosis. In the Cotton test, the talus is translated within the mortise in the medial-lateral plane and, similarly, increased translation and pain with this maneuver indicate a positive test result. In the relatively newly described crossed-leg test, the seated patient positions the mid-fibula of his or her injured leg on the knee of the uninvolved leg, and pushes the knee on the affected leg toward the ground; pain felt in the syndesmosis demonstrates a positive test result. This test is effectively a variation of the squeeze test, but may have the added advantage that there will tend to be an additional external rotation force on the ankle by gravity. Among the common clinical tests, only the external rotation test has been proved to correlate with syndesmotic injury and with more protracted duration until resumption of preinjury function.[38,39]

IMAGING

Standard radiographs of the ankle, comprising weight-bearing anteroposterior (AP), mortise, and lateral views, should be the first set of investigations obtained for a patient with clinically suspected syndesmosis injury. In these views, assessment may be made of the relationship between the distal tibia and fibula, and the presence of malleolar fractures and bony avulsions of the anterior or posterior tibia, which are present in up to 50% of all syndesmosis injuries.[40] Occasionally complete tibia-fibula AP and lateral views are necessary to identify a possible Maisonneuve fracture. In chronic injuries, there may be a synostosis between the tibia and fibula.

Good-quality radiographs and consistent positioning are vital in syndesmosis injuries, as millimeter values are disputed in its diagnosis. Diastasis is detected on the AP and mortise radiographs by a widened tibiofibular clear space measuring 6 mm or greater, and a reduced tibiofibular overlap measuring less than 6 mm on the AP radiograph or measuring 1 mm or less on the mortise radiograph (**Fig. 3**). Of these, the most reliable radiographic landmark in detecting early widening of the syndesmosis is the tibiofibular clear space seen on both AP and mortise views.[41] Individual

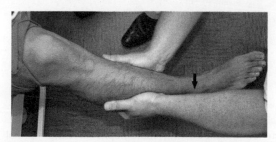

Fig. 1. Squeeze test. (*arrow* indicates the site of pain when performing the test).

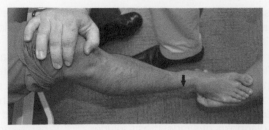

Fig. 2. External rotation test. (*arrow* indicates the site of pain when performing the test).

variability and gender-specific differences exist, which complicates matters. A tibiofibular clear space of less than 5.2 mm in females or 6.47 mm in males, and a tibiofibular overlap of greater than 2.1 mm in females or 5.7 mm in males, should be considered normal.[42] Because of these differences, comparison radiographs of the contralateral ankle may be valuable in reducing confusion in diagnosis.

When diastasis is frank, it may be readily seen on routine radiographs. However, when diastasis is latent, some investigators have advocated the use of stress radiographs as the next step in exposing the injury. External rotation or lateral shift forces are applied to the ankle to reproduce widening of the mortise and posterior displacement of the fibula.[27] However, stress radiography has been shown to have a high false-negative rate, as many syndesmotic disruptions are not obvious on stress views but are only later detected at arthroscopy, and should therefore be used cautiously and only as an adjunct to diagnosis.[26]

Arthrography was previously widely used to visualize the distal tibiofibular joint, and had a reported rate of 90% sensitivity and 67% specificity.[43] Bone scanning of the ankle with technetium-99m pyrophosphate can demonstrate trauma through increased uptake with a reported rate of 100% sensitivity and 71% specificity.[22] Ultrasound scanning (**Fig. 4**) may be used to visualize injuries to the ligament in static and dynamic modes in the clinical setting, and this method has a reported sensitivity of

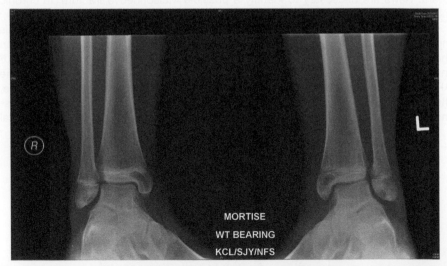

Fig. 3. Anteroposterior weight-bearing radiographs showing normal right ankle and syndesmosis injury with reduced tibiofibular overlap of left ankle.

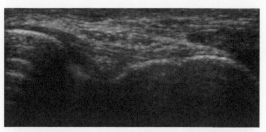

Fig. 4. Ultrasonogram showing the normal fibrillar pattern of the AITFL.

67%, but is very user dependent.[44] These techniques have value but have largely been replaced by CT and magnetic resonance imaging (MRI).

MRI and CT are currently the imaging modalities of choice in most centers. MRI allows accurate delineation of the syndesmotic ligaments.[45] The AITFL and PITFL are identified on axial and coronal sequences as hypointense, thin structures at the level of the tibial plafond and talar dome (**Fig. 5**). Compared with intraoperative arthroscopic examinations of the syndesmosis, MRI has been proved to equate well, with reported sensitivities of 100% for detecting AITFL and PITFL tears, and specificities of 93% and 100% for AITFL and PITFL tears, respectively (**Figs. 6** and **7**).[46] Its wide field of view allows detection of concomitant injuries, with no radiation burden to the patient (**Fig. 8**). Disadvantages of MRI include that it incurs the highest cost and that the relatively thick slices means that small avulsion fragments or loose bodies may be missed. CT provides excellent bone detail, and the thin slices allow for

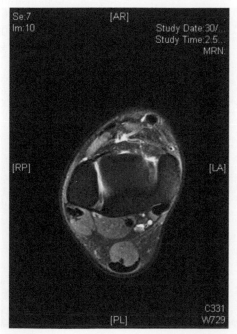

Fig. 5. Axial proton-density fat-saturated MRI scan showing normal appearance of the AITFL and PITFL.

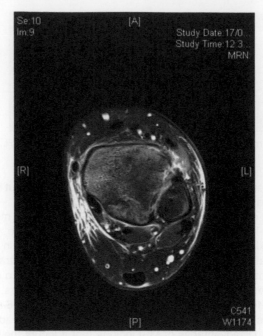

Fig. 6. Axial proton-density fat-saturated sequence showing acute tears of the AITFL and PITFL.

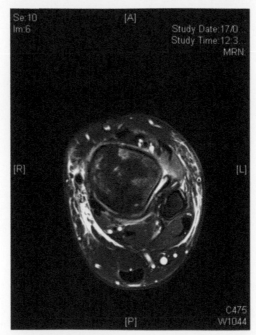

Fig. 7. Axial proton-density fat-saturated sequence showing displaced free end of torn AITFL.

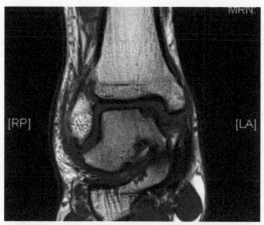

Fig. 8. T1-weighted coronal MRI scan showing concomitant osteochondral lesion of the talar dome.

associated bony avulsions to be appreciated. In addition, 3-dimensional images of the mortise can be reconstructed using CT. CT imaging has also improved the accuracy in detection of diastases of as small as 1 mm, not previously identifiable on plain radiographs.[47]

CLASSIFICATION

Syndesmosis injuries have been classified both chronologically and radiographically. The chronologic approach is standard to any traumatic musculoskeletal condition, and helps to guide treatment. Syndesmosis injuries may be divided into acute (within first 3 weeks of injury), subacute (3 weeks to 3 months), and chronic (beyond 3 months) injuries.

In the system by Edwards and DeLee,[31] traumatic syndesmotic diastases are classified into latent or frank groups. Within the frank diastasis group, 4 further subdivisions were made: Type I is frank diastasis with lateral subluxation of the fibula without fracture; Type II is when the fibula is plastically deformed in addition to lateral subluxated; Type III involves posterior subluxation or dislocation of the fibula; and Type IV involves superior wedging of the talus into the mortise. The latter 2 entities are exceptionally rare, and hence this classification system has been thought to be of questionable clinical relevance by some practitioners.[8]

The West Point Ankle Grading System proposed by Gerber and colleagues[7] classifies pure ligamentous syndesmosis injuries into 3 grades based on the degree of instability, and the criteria used for its determination are ability to bear weight, the extent of the edema, the localization of tenderness, response to provocative stress tests, and evidence of radiographic widening observed. Grade I suggests no instability, Grade II suggests some evidence of instability, and Grade III indicates definite instability. Each increasing grade correlates with progressive disruption of the syndesmotic ligaments: Grade I, partial tear of AITFL; Grade II, tear of AITFL and partial tear of IOL; and Grade III, complete tear of syndesmotic ligaments. As these grades may be thought of as a spectrum of tears instead of true categories in themselves, it may be difficult to distinguish between, for example, Grade I and Grade II tears. In this same study, functional treatment of Grade I and Grade II injuries did not show differences in their outcomes.

At present there is no classification system that allows clear definition of the degree of injury, guidance of treatment, or prediction of outcome. Clinicians base their decisions on the signs and symptoms of individual patients, their level of activity and expectations, and an interpretation of the severity of the diastasis as revealed by imaging studies. One should be mindful too that congenital forms of diastasis exist, but this topic is outside the scope of this article.

NATURAL HISTORY AND ASSOCIATED INJURIES

For elite athletes, syndesmosis injuries may result in time loss from practice or competition and residual morbidity caused by persistent symptoms. The time loss varies from one study to another. In one article studying the effect of this injury on professional football players, the average time lost was reported as 2.5 weeks, 11.7 practices, or 1.4 games.[48] In comparison, collegiate football players in another study required an average of 31 days before return to full activity.[49] The number of days missed from competition was found to correlate with the length of interosseous tenderness. Persistent stiffness and pain during push-off are possible sequelae. At the end of a follow-up period of 47 months on 44 collegiate football players, most players were in the category with no symptoms or mild symptoms; however, the remaining 6 players still experienced moderate symptoms. Patients with prolonged recovery periods were observed to have radiographic evidence of ossification of the interosseous membrane. Synostosis of the ankle syndesmosis is thought to cause protracted symptoms of pain and stiffness, leading to disability.[25] A retrospective study of football players with syndesmosis injuries found that the presence of synostosis was implicated in prolonging the recovery time.[49] As the etiology of this sequelae is not yet fully understood, preventive measures have yet to be identified. The prevalence of synostosis was found to be higher when bioabsorbable implants were used for fixation.[50] The increased use of MRI as a diagnostic tool has highlighted the multitude of concomitant injuries not previously demonstrated, and empowers the surgeon with a more tailored approach with which to address these injuries. The rate of associated injuries is high: anterior talofibular ligament injuries 83%, acute bone bruises 78%, acute talar dome osteochondral injuries 48%, and osteoarthritis in chronic injuries 19%.[12] In short, syndesmosis injuries run the gamut from simple isolated sprains to frank diastases with fractures and a host of other potential injuries. The presentation is variable, making accurate prognostication of these injuries difficult with regard to time lost and ankle pain or dysfunction.

TREATMENT
Acute Syndesmotic Injury: Conservative Treatment

Syndesmosis sprains without diastasis are generally and adequately managed with a conservative course of treatment. In athletes, the key consideration is in tailoring a program unique to their specific need, with the aim of returning them to their preinjury level of function in a safe and timely manner. In treating a patient conservatively there are many questions that need to be considered from the outset: the need for immobilization, the necessity for weight-bearing restriction, time lines for healing, assessments that may determine healing, and ultimately, time for safe and effective return to sports. The progress of rehabilitation is largely steered by the individual's response to therapy, but in general a 3-phase approach may be used as a broad framework to conservative management of these injuries.[7,32,51] The first phase is an acute phase directed at protecting the injured ankle and limiting the inflammatory response and pain, through the first-aid formula, RICE (Rest, Ice, Compression, and

Elevation of the limb). At this stage, the treating surgeon or physician is confronted with issues of immobilization and weight bearing, both of which pertain to protection of the ankle joint. Williams and colleagues[33] proposed immobilization of the ankle in patients with severe injuries, significant pain, and muscle deactivation; they also recommended that the level of weight bearing be dependent on the severity of injury and symptoms, but that in general weight bearing should be assisted until normal gait has resumed, thence to progress without unwarranted delay to avoid complications associated with prolonged disuse. The second phase is a subacute phase that involves joint mobilization, strength training, and restoration of basic ankle functions. In the third phase, the athlete progresses to advanced training of proprioception for return to sports through sports-specific drills, such as cutting, pivoting, shuffling, and jumping, that require reactive neuromuscular control. It is difficult to establish when an athlete is able to return to sports, and this decision is made through careful consideration of the patient's report, functional testing results, and clinical examination. Conservative treatment of syndesmosis sprains has an overall reported rate of 86% to 100% good to excellent outcomes, and almost all cases achieve full return to sports.[6,7,52]

Acute Syndesmotic Injury: Surgical Treatment

In general, acute syndesmotic injuries with frank or latent diastases are indications for surgical treatment. There are exceptions to this guideline. The first is the patient whose latent diastasis has achieved closed anatomic reduction of the fibula documented on CT or MRI. The second is the patient whose frank diastases with posterior subluxation or dislocation of the fibula (Edwards and DeLee Type III), or with superior subluxation or dislocation of the talus into the mortise (Edwards and DeLee Type IV), has evidence of reduction having been successfully achieved after closed longitudinal traction. These injuries may be managed conservatively as described in the previous section. Nevertheless, the authors and other groups recommend a lowered threshold for surgery in professional athletes who fall into these groups.[33,53]

Pure ligamentous diastasis of the distal tibiofibular joint is more common than osteoligamentous avulsion from the anterior tubercle of the fibula or distal tibia in adults. Whereas indirect reduction and percutaneous fixation is commonly performed for pure ligamentous injuries, some investigators recommend that the distal tibiofibular joint be approached through an anterolateral approach.[8,22,54] This approach enables the space to be inspected directly and be cleared of any osteofibrocartilaginous debris that may hinder anatomic reduction. In this approach, care must be taken not to traumatize the branches of the superficial peroneal nerve; hence blunt dissection of the subcutaneous layer is advised. If the medial clear space is persistently widened and accurate reduction cannot be achieved by this approach alone, a separate medial incision may be necessary to explore this space and free it from interposed deltoid ligament (with repair or reattachment of the deep deltoid) or capsular tissue. The evidence for direct suture repair of the torn deltoid ligament, however, is not yet clear.[8] The distal tibiofibular joint is reduced using bimalleolar reduction clamps while repeated fluoroscopic examinations ensure the fibula is properly positioned before definitive fixation.

The fixation of pure ligamentous syndesmosis injuries may be rigid or semirigid. The restored distal tibiofibular joint may be fixed rigidly by way of a transsyndesmosis screw, classically placed proximal and parallel to the ankle joint. Although screw fixation is a standard and common form of fixation, the existing data show controversies with regard to various aspects of screw fixation (see later discussion). As already mentioned, physiologic motion occurs between the distal tibia and fibula in rotational and proximal-distal planes, thus semirigid fixation may be theoretically more desirable than rigid fixation. Suture-buttons (**Fig. 9**) have been tensioned across the syndesmosis to maintain its dynamic relationship, with promising results. Seitz and colleagues[55] found the suture-button to be comparable with a 4.5-mm screw fixed across 4 cortices. In a cadaveric study, Thornes and colleagues[56] compared the Suture-Endobutton construct with syndesmosis screw fixation, and found that the Suture-Endobutton at least paralleled the performance of screw fixation. The clinical trial by Thornes and colleagues[57] published 2 years later showed that the Suture-Endobutton was associated with shorter rehabilitation, faster return to work, and no complications. However, as Thornes was the inventor of the Suture-Endobutton, a potential conflict of interest may affect the interpretation of the results. By contrast, a cadaveric biomechanical study by Forsythe and colleagues[58] reported the inability of the suture-button to maintain adequate syndesmotic reduction when compared with the metallic screw, as it failed to withstand the forces imparted on the ankle, particularly rotational forces.

If a sufficiently large fragment is avulsed from the Chaput or Wagstaffe tubercle, it should be fixed with a small screw and, if possible, reinforced with the addition of a washer. If the osseous fragment is too small for fixation, it may be excised and the ligament repaired using suture anchors.

Syndesmosis injury occurs in up to 13% of patients with ankle fractures.[59,60] It is most commonly seen in Weber C fractures, but the surgeon must be aware of its occasional presence in the Weber B variety. If an associated malleolar fracture is present, anatomic fixation of the fracture is paramount to enable proper reduction of the distal tibiofibular joint. Malleolar fracture malreduction is unforgiving and will result in unsatisfactory reduction of the syndesmosis, which will in turn affect the outcome. Significant correlations have been proved to exist between (1) the adequacy of reduction of the syndesmosis and late arthritis, (2) the accuracy of initial reduction of the syndesmosis and late stability of the syndesmosis, (3) late stability of the syndesmosis and the final outcome, and (4) the adequacy of the reduction of the lateral malleolus and that of the syndesmosis.[61] Syndesmosis malreduction was shown by Kennedy and colleagues[62] to be associated with poor outcomes, consistent with findings documented years earlier by Chissell and Jones,[63] who demonstrated that a syndesmosis width of greater than 1.5 mm was associated with unacceptable outcome at 2 to 8 years' follow-up. In fact, a recent article showed that reduction of the syndesmosis was the only significant predictor of functional outcome after transsyndesmosis screw fixation in ankle fractures.[64] A review of CT scans reported that syndesmosis reduction was usually inadequate.[65] Underreduction of the syndesmosis was undetected in 24% of cases despite good-quality radiographs and fluoroscopy.[66,67] Several studies advocate postoperative CT scanning of both ankles to allow early detection of incongruence that may require early revision.[66,68] The pursuit of the perfect mortise is warranted, as the existing data clearly point to necessary anatomic restoration of

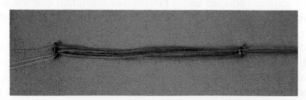

Fig. 9. Example of a suture fixation device (Syndesmosis TightRope; Arthrex, Naples, FL) used in the treatment of syndesmosis injuries.

the syndesmosis for prevention of late syndesmotic instability and development of posttraumatic arthritis.

Multiple studies have attempted to outline instances when syndesmosis screw fixation may be omitted in ankle fractures. Some practitioners suggested that the diastasis screw fixation was used needlessly in many patients, but the unnecessary fixation did not compromise their final functional results.[63,64,69] Factors that should be considered in the preoperative planning of these cases are medial ankle injury, be it the integrity of the deltoid ligament or presence of medial malleolus fracture, and level of fibular fracture.

The plastically deformed fibula, seen in the younger age group, may pose a challenge to reduction. Although rare, the surgeon must be aware that it may block complete reduction and that a proximal osteotomy of the fibula may be needed if reduction is problematic before syndesmosis stabilization.[31]

In general, the literature supports an initial period of non–weight bearing followed by progressive weight bearing postoperatively. The syndesmosis screw should be removed only after healing has occurred. Recommendations for the timing of screw removal range from as early as 6 weeks postoperatively to later than 12 weeks postoperatively. Screws that are left permanently in situ risk osteolysis or breakage when the patient regains normal motion and function of the ankle joint.[70–72] The arguments that pertain to the postoperative regimen are discussed later this article.

Chronic Syndesmosis Injury

The patient with chronic syndesmosis injury often experiences vague symptoms. Presenting complaints include persistent ankle pain with sensation of giving way typically felt when walking on uneven ground, stiffness and limited dorsiflexion, and inability to achieve a preinjury level of function.[10,73] There may be persistent tenderness and swelling in the anterolateral aspect of the ankle. The clinical suspicion is proved with weight bearing and positive stress radiographs of the ankle. It is useful to make a comparison with the normal side. As with acute injuries, the distal tibiofibular bony relationship is seen most clearly on CT imaging. Malreduced malleolar fractures, bony avulsions, and the presence of synostosis in the distal tibiofibular joint may also be assessed with accuracy for surgical planning.

As emphasized earlier, chronic injuries render the syndesmosis biomechanically inferior because of instability, and may result in arthritis. Despite its problems, the literature is comparatively scarce regarding management options for chronic syndesmosis ruptures.

Treatment performed for symptomatic relief only, without restoring stability of the joint, has been demonstrated to be a useful and uncomplicated option. In a study by Ogilvie-Harris and colleagues,[9] all of their patients with chronic injuries who were treated with arthroscopic debridement of the torn IOL and chondroplasty reported short-term relief of symptoms. It has been suggested that the primary generators of pain in chronic syndesmotic injury are soft-tissue hypertrophy that impinges against the lateral talar dome and adhesions within the syndesmosis that limit motion. Arthroscopic excision of these structures, implicated as sources of pain, has been shown to provide significant functional improvement in studies by Han and colleagues[74] and Pritsch and colleagues.[75]

For the elite athlete, it is clear that the restoration of stability is a vital part of the management strategy, in addition to attaining symptomatic relief. Many case reports have detailed a variety of operative options for late reconstruction of the chronically injured syndesmosis. In an early article, lag screw fixation was used successfully to treat recurrent ankle sprains in the subacute and chronic stages.[76] Another article described the use of a 6.5-mm cancellous screw to engage 4 cortices across the chronically unstable syndesmosis.[11] Wolf and Amendola[53] reported on the outcome of their treatment of athletically active patients with chronic syndesmosis injuries without diastasis or fracture by arthroscopic debridement and percutaneous transsyndesmotic screw fixation for 8 to 10 weeks. At a minimum of 6 months, results were rated as excellent in 14%, good in 71%, and fair in 14%. In another method, the attenuated AITFL was retensioned by medial and proximal mobilization, and refixation by way of a 0.7 × 0.7-cm bone block fixed using a screw, with additional use of a quadricortical syndesmotic screw. All patients improved, and none complained of ankle instability at a mean follow-up time of 45 months.[10]

Reconstruction of the chronically torn syndesmotic ligaments aims to restore the physiologic dynamic relationship of the distal tibiofibular joint. In an early article, Castaing and colleagues[77] described the use of autogenous peroneus brevis tendon for the reconstruction of the AITFL and PITFL. Later, this technique underwent modification to more closely match the syndesmotic anatomy and to enhance its stability. In this technically demanding procedure, the peroneal longus tendon is used for ligamentoplasty. It is split and weaved through 1 bone channel in the distal tibia parallel to the fibular incisura and through 2 channels in the distal fibula at 45° to each other, to recreate the AITFL, IOL, and PITFL complex. At 18 months' follow-up, all but 1 of the 16 patients had relief of pain and instability.[73]

Ankle syndesmosis arthrodesis is an excellent option as a salvage procedure in cases of painful arthritis with chronic syndesmotic instability. It is used as last resort when other options have failed or can no longer be considered. Pena and Coetzee[25] recommended arthrodesis after 6 months and only if significant incongruence is demonstrated on CT images. In their description, the syndesmosis fusion site is stripped and packed with bone graft, and fixation is achieved using 2 syndesmosis screws and a plate. Weight bearing is allowed only after radiographic fusion is seen, usually at the eighth or tenth week after surgery.

Controversies in Surgical Treatment

Fixation of the syndesmosis is traditionally and commonly done with the foot maximally dorsiflexed. It is understood that this position allows the widest anterior part of the talus to engage into the mortise, thus avoiding overcompression of the mortise and subsequent postoperative limited ankle range of movement.[78] This practice has more recently been shown not to be mandatory in a recent cadaveric study, which concluded that the position of the foot during syndesmosis fixation does not affect the postoperative range of ankle motion.[79]

Another debated topic is the number of screws used, the size of screws used, and the number of cortices fixed. Traditionally 1 or 2 metallic screws are used to engage across 3 or 4 cortices to stabilize the syndesmosis in a reduced position to facilitate healing. One screw may be sufficient in a Weber C fracture that is fixed anatomically, but an additional screw may be beneficial in an acute isolated diastasis without fracture or with a Maisonneuve fracture where the fibula fracture is not primarily fixed. Occasionally in the latter, a 2-hole one-third tubular plate is used as a washer for the screws to maximize compression of the syndesmosis joint.[22] Tricortical fixation is biomechanically adequate to fix the distal tibiofibular joint in position. By contrast, quadricortical fixation is beneficial when screw breakage occurs, as direct access to the broken fragment from the tibial end will enable its easy retrieval. Cortical screw sizes of 4.5 mm and 3.5 mm have been used for fixation, although the optimal screw size has not been defined. In the authors' practice, in cases of diastasis associated with a high fibular fracture, the syndesmosis is reduced using a pair of pelvic reduction clamps while repeatedly checking that the anatomy has been restored using fluoro-scopic guidance. Once it is satisfactory, 2 metallic 3.5-mm cortical screws placed parallel to and 2 to 4 cm proximal to the ankle joint line are used, entering from the posterolateral aspect of the distal fibula and directed 30° anterior into the tibia. In cases where the fibula fracture is lower, the fracture is fixed anatomically before the syndesmosis is tested intraoperatively for instability by pulling laterally on the distal fibula using a bone hook. If widening is demonstrated, transsyndesmotic fixation with a single screw will suffice. The transsyndesmotic screw does not lag the syndes-mosis joint, but functions as a positioning or neutralization screw.

In general, several weeks of non–weight bearing is recommended during healing while the screw is in place. It is difficult to determine precisely when healing is complete, when the screw may be removed safely, and when weight bearing should commence. Each case varies to a certain extent depending on the individual's factors. Some investigators advise removal of the screw at the earliest 3 months postopera-tively, and warn about the risk of fixation failure if removal is done prematurely within 6 to 8 weeks postoperatively.[22,80,81] Others allow graduated weight bearing starting at 6 weeks postoperatively with the screw in situ, with average time for removal at 8 to 10 weeks.[33] It is sensible to delay screw removal and return to sports for patients who are heavy, poorly compliant, or have pes planovalgus, as these individuals have an inherent tendency for external rotation of the foot and ankle.[33]

Bioabsorbable screws have increased in popularity because their use negates the need for hardware removal, while providing stability and clinical results equivalent to those of metallic screws.[82–85] The main and widely documented drawback of the biodegradable polylactic and polyglycolic screws is that they may incite local inflam-matory and osteolytic foreign-body adverse reactions, which can manifest as sterile abscesses or cysts.[83,86–88] Another practical issue is the challenge faced in the extrac-tion of a screw, for example for infection, while it is in its half-dissolved state.

In cases of athletes with high ankle sprain without fracture where the fibula length is maintained, the authors recommend a tightrope stabilization. The postoperative regime involves an Aircast boot for 4 weeks with the patient non–weight bearing for the first 2 weeks, then weight bearing as tolerated. Each case is monitored by a phys-iotherapist, but in general running in a straight line (ie, on a treadmill) can be expected after 6 weeks, after which cutting and turning is introduced as the athlete feels able to.

Controversies prevail with regard to whether nonoperative treatment or early surgery should be recommended in those whose syndesmosis injuries do not demon-strate widening on radiographs. Whichever method is used, it must be able to achieve the immediate aim of obtaining and maintaining anatomic reduction of the syndes-motic joint until it heals. In so doing, the long-term problems of late pain and instability that debilitate those who have chronic syndesmosis injuries may be averted.

SUMMARY

Syndesmosis injury is a term that encompasses any form of trauma to the distal tibio-fibular joint. Appreciation of the injury and the ability to diagnose the mild sprains that more commonly affect the sporting population, compared with the more obvious frank diastases with associated fractures, have improved. The treating physician or surgeon must maintain a high index of suspicion and consciously look for this injury when faced with an injured athlete, through a combination of meticulous and relevant history taking, clinical examination, and imaging. One must avoid missing this diagnosis, as poor management will result in unacceptable disability to the athlete in the short and long term. The aim when treating elite athletes is to return them to their specific preinjury level of function in as safe a manner as possible and without undue delay. To achieve this, the first prerequisite for successful treatment is anatomic restoration of the syndesmosis that must be maintained throughout the duration of treatment until healing is complete. There is greater awareness that a large proportion of treated injuries actually remain malreduced, and therefore early postoperative CT imaging and revision via an open reduction, if necessary, are increasingly being advocated. Current understanding dictates that acute sprains may be managed nonoperatively or with a tightrope, with acute frank diastases or acute occult injuries that cannot be reduced in a closed fashion being stabilized operatively. It is interesting that almost every aspect of surgical treatment of syndesmosis injuries is fraught with controversies. In view of the high incidence of these injuries among elite athletes and the challenges faced by the treating practitioner, further research is required to more reliably give a prognosis following these injuries, and to determine which of the different treatment options is best.

REFERENCES

1. Hopkinson WJ, St Pierre P, Ryan JB, et al. Syndesmosis sprains of the ankle. Foot Ankle 1990;10(6):325–30.
2. Boytim MJ, Fischer DA, Neumann L. Syndesmotic ankle sprains. Am J Sports Med 1991;19(3):294–8.
3. Wright RW, Barile RJ, Surprenant DA, et al. Ankle syndesmosis sprains in National Hockey League players. Am J Sports Med 2004;32:1941–5.
4. Wuest TK. Injuries to the distal lower extremity syndesmosis. J Am Acad Orthop Surg 1997;5:172–81.
5. Ward DW. Syndesmotic ankle sprain in a recreational hockey player. J Manipulative Physiol Ther 1994;17:385–94.
6. Taylor DC, Bassett FH. Syndesmosis ankle sprains: diagnosing the injury and aiding recovery. Physician Sportsmed 1993;21(12):39–46.
7. Gerber JP, Williams GN, Scoville CR, et al. Persistent disability associated with ankle sprains: a prospective examination of an athletic population. Foot Ankle Int 1998;19:653–60.
8. Rammelt S, Zwipp H, Grass R. Injuries to the distal tibiofibular syndesmosis. Foot Ankle Clin 2008;13:611–33.
9. Ogilvie-Harris DJ, Gilbart MK, Chorney K. Chronic pain following ankle sprains in athletes: the role of arthroscopic surgery. Arthroscopy 1997;13(5):564–74.
10. Beumer A, Heijboer RP, Fontijne WP, et al. Late reconstruction of the anterior distal tibiofibular syndesmosis: good outcome in 9 patients. Acta Orthop Scand 2000;71(5):519–21.
11. Harper MC. Delayed reduction and stabilization of the tibiofibular syndesmosis. Foot Ankle Int 2001;22(1):15–8.
12. Brown KW, Morrison WB, Schweitzer ME, et al. MRI findings associated with distal tibiofibular syndesmosis injury. AJR Am J Roentgenol 2004;182:131–6.
13. Bromfield W. Chirurgical observations and cases, vol. 2. London: Cadell; 1773.
14. Quenu E. Du diastasis de l'articulation tibio-péronière inferieure. Rev Chir (Paris) 1907;36:62–90 [in French].
15. Sauer HD, Jungfer E, Jungbluth KH. Experimentelle Untersuchungen zur Reißfestigkeit des Bandapparates am menschlichen Sprunggelenk. Hefte Unfallheilkd 1978;131:37–42 [in German].
16. Rasmussen O. Stability of the ankle joint: analysis of the function and traumatology of the ankle ligaments. Acta Orthop Scand 1985;211:1–75.

17. Kelikian H, Kelikian AS. Disorders of the ankle. Philadelphia: W.B. Saunders; 1985.
18. Sarrafian SK. Anatomy of the foot and ankle: descriptive, topographic, functional. Philadelphia: JB Lippincott; 1983.
19. Bartonicek J. Anatomy of the tibiofibular syndesmosis and its clinical relevance. Surg Radiol Anat 2003;25(5–6):379–86.
20. Lutz W. Zur Struktur der unteren Tibiofibularverbindung und der Membrana interossea cruris. Zeitschrift für Anatomie und Entwicklungsgeschichte 1942;111: 315–21 [in German].
21. Höcker K, Pachucki A. The fibular incisure of the tibia. The cross-sectional position of the fibula in distal syndesmosis. Unfallchirurg 1989;92(8):401–6 [in German].
22. Espinosa N, Smerek JP, Myerson M. Acute and chronic syndesmosis injuries: pathomechanicsms, diagnosis and management. Foot Ankle Clin 2006;11: 639–57.
23. Ebraheim NA, Lu J, Yang H, et al. The fibular incisure of the tibia on CT scan: a cadaver study. Foot Ankle Int 1998;19(5):318–21.
24. Elgafy H, Semaan HB, Blessinger B, et al. Computed tomography of normal distal tibiofibular syndesmosis. Skeletal Radiol 2010;39(6):559–64.
25. Pena FA, Coetzee JC. Ankle syndesmosis injuries. Foot Ankle Clin 2006;11: 35–50.
26. Ogilvie-Harris DJ, Reed SC. Disruption of the ankle syndesmosis: diagnosis and treatment by arthroscopic surgery. Arthroscopy 1994;10:561–8.
27. Xenos JS, Hopkinson WJ, Mulligan ME, et al. The tibiofibular syndesmosis: evaluation of the ligamentous structures, methods of fixation, and radiographic assessment. J Bone Joint Surg Am 1995;77:847–56.
28. Ramsey PL, Hamilton W. Changes in tibiotalar area of contact caused by lateral talar shift. J Bone Joint Surg Am 1976;58:356–7.
29. Zindrick MR, Hopkins DE, Knight GW, et al. The effect of lateral talar shift upon the biomechanics of the ankle joint. Orthopaedic Transactions 1985;9: 332–3.
30. Thordarson DB, Motamed S, Hedman T, et al. The effect of fibular malreduction on contact pressures in an ankle fracture malunion model. J Bone Joint Surg Am 1997;79(12):1809–15.
31. Edwards GS Jr, DeLee JC. Ankle diastasis without fracture. Foot Ankle 1984;4(6): 305–12.
32. Nussbaum ED, Hosea TM, Sieler SD, et al. Prospective evaluation of syndesmotic ankle sprains without diastasis. Am J Sports Med 2001;29(1):31–5.
33. Williams GN, Jones MH, Amendola A. Syndesmotic ankle sprains in athletes. Am J Sports Med 2007;35(7):1197–207.
34. Cedell CA. Ankle lesions. Acta Orthop Scand 1975;46:425–45.
35. Mulligan E. Evaluation and management of ankle syndesmosis injuries. Phys Ther Sport 2011;12:57–69.
36. Beumer A, van Hemert WL, Swierstra BA, et al. A biomechanical evaluation of clinical stress tests for syndesmotic ankle instability. Foot Ankle Int 2003;24: 358–63.
37. Kiter E, Bozkurt M. The crossed-leg test for examination of ankle syndesmosis injuries. Foot Ankle Int 2005;26:187–8.
38. Beumer A, Swierstra BA, Mulder PG. Clinical diagnosis of syndesmotic ankle instability: evaluation of stress tests behind the curtains. Acta Orthop Scand 2002;73(6):667–9.

39. Alonso A, Khoury L, Adams R. Clinical tests for ankle syndesmosis injury: reliability and prediction of return to function. J Orthop Sports Phys Ther 1998; 27(4):276–84.
40. Frey C. Ankle sprains. Instr Course Lect 2001;50:515–20.
41. Harper MC, Keller TS. A radiographic evaluation of the tibiofibular syndesmosis. Foot Ankle 1989;10:156–60.
42. Ostrum RF, de Meo P, Subramanian R. A critical analysis of the anterior-posterior radiographic anatomy of the ankle syndesmosis. Foot Ankle Int 1995;16(3): 128–31.
43. Wrazidlo VW, Karl E, Koch K. Die arthrographische diagnostik der vorderen syndesmosenrupturam oberen sprunggelenk. [Arthrographic diagnosis of rupture of the anterior syndesmosis of the upper ankle joint]. Rofo 1988;148:492–7 [in German].
44. Milz P, Milz S, Steinborn M, et al. Lateral ankle ligaments and tibiofibular syndesmosis. 13 MHz high-frequency sonography and MRI compared in 20 patients. Acta Orthop Scand 1998;69:51–5.
45. Muhle C, Frank LR, Rand T, et al. Tibiofibular syndesmosis: high-resolution MRI using a local gradient coil. J Comput Assist Tomogr 1998;22:938–44.
46. Takao M, Ochi M, Oae K, et al. Diagnosis of a tear of the tibiofibular syndesmosis: the role of arthroscopy of the ankle. J Bone Joint Surg Br 2003;85: 324–9.
47. Ebraheim NA, Lu J, Yang H, et al. Radiographic and CT evaluation of tibiofibular syndesmotic diastasis: a cadaver study. Foot Ankle Int 1997;18:693–8.
48. Guise ER. Rotational ligamentous injuries to the ankle in football. Am J Sports Med 1976;4:1–6.
49. Taylor DC, Englehardt DL, Bassett FH 3rd. Syndesmosis sprains of the ankle: the influence of heterotopic ossification. Am J Sports Med 1992;20:146–50.
50. Bostman OM. Distal tibiofibular synostosis after malleolar fractures treated using absorbable implants. Foot Ankle 1993;14:38–43.
51. Brosky T, Nyland J, Nitz A, et al. The ankle ligaments: consideration of syndesmotic injury and implications for rehabilitation. J Orthop Sports Phys Ther 1995; 21:197–205.
52. Amendola A, Williams G, Foster D. Evidence-based approach to treatment of acute traumatic syndesmosis (high ankle) sprains. Sports Med Arthrosc 2006; 14(4):232–6.
53. Wolf BR, Amendola A. Syndesmosis injuries in the athlete: when and how to operate. Curr Opin Orthop 2002;31:151–4.
54. Clanton TO, Paul P. Syndesmosis injuries in athletes. Foot Ankle Clin 2002;7: 529–49.
55. Seitz WH Jr, Bachner EJ, Abram LJ, et al. Repair of the tibiofibular syndesmosis with a flexible implant. J Orthop Trauma 1991;5(1):78–82.
56. Thornes B, Walsh A, Hislop M, et al. Suture-endobutton fixation of ankle tibiofibular diastasis: a cadaveric study. Foot Ankle Int 2003;24:142–6.
57. Thornes B, Shannon F, Guiney AM, et al. Suture-button syndesmosis fixation: accelerated rehabilitation and improved outcomes. Clin Orthop Relat Res 2005; 431:207–12.
58. Forsythe K, Freedman KB, Stover MD, et al. Comparison of a novel fiberwire-button construct versus metallic screw fixation in a syndesmotic injury model. Foot Ankle Int 2008;29:49–54.
59. Lindsjo U. Operative treatment of ankle fractures. Acta Orthop Scand 1981; 189(Suppl 189):1–131.

60. Court-Brown CM, McBirnie J, Wilson G. Adult ankle fractures: an increasing problem? Acta Orthop Scand 1998;69:43–7.
61. Leeds HC, Ehrlich MG. Instability of the distal tibiofibular syndesmosis after bimalleolar and trimalleolar ankle fractures. J Bone Joint Surg Am 1984;66: 490–503.
62. Kennedy JG, Soffe KE, Dalla Vedova P, et al. Evaluation of the syndesmotic screw in low Weber C ankle fractures. J Orthop Trauma 2000;14(5):359–66.
63. Chissell HR, Jones J. The influence of a diastasis screw on the outcome of Weber type-C ankle fractures. J Bone Joint Surg Br 1995;77(3):435–8.
64. Weening B, Bhandari M. Predictors of functional outcome following transsyndesmotic screw fixation of ankle fractures. J Orthop Trauma 2005;19(2):102–8.
65. Pottorff GT, Kaye RA. CT assessment of syndesmosis in Weber C ankle fractures. Paper presented at the American Orthopaedic Foot and Ankle Society Specialty Day. Washington, DC, February 23, 1992.
66. Barthel S, Grass R, Zwipp H. Stellenwert der Computertomographie bei der Evaluierung operativ versorgter Sprunggelenksfrakturen. Hefte Unfalchir 2002;284: 235–6 [in German].
67. Gardner MJ, Demetrakopoulos D, Briggs SM, et al. Malreduction of the tibiofibular syndesmosis in ankle fractures. Foot Ankle Int 2006;27(10):788–92.
68. Vasarhelyi A, Lubitz J, Gierer P, et al. Detection of fibular torsional deformities after surgery for ankle fractures with a novel CT method. Foot Ankle Int 2006; 27(12):1115–21.
69. Yamaguchi K, Martin CH, Boden SD, et al. Operative treatment of syndesmotic disruptions without use of a syndesmotic screw: a prospective clinical study. Foot Ankle Int 1994;15(8):407–14.
70. Heim U. Malleolar fractures. Unfallheilkunde 1983;86(6):248–58 [in German].
71. Grass R, Herzmann K, Biewener A, et al. Injuries of the distal tibiofibular syndesmosis. Unfallchirurg 2000;103:520–32 [in German].
72. Kaye RA. Stabilization of ankle syndesmosis injuries with a syndesmosis screw. Foot Ankle 1989;9(6):290–3.
73. Grass R, Rammelt S, Biewener A, et al. Peroneus longus ligamentoplasty for chronic instability of the distal tibiofibular syndesmosis. Foot Ankle Int 2003; 24(5):392–7.
74. Han SH, Lee JW, Kim S, et al. Chronic tibiofibular syndesmosis injury: the diagnostic efficiency of magnetic resonance imaging and comparative analysis of operative treatment. Foot Ankle Int 2007;28(3):336–42.
75. Pritsch M, Lokiec F, Sali M, et al. Adhesions of distal tibiofibular syndesmosis: a cause of chronic ankle pain after fracture. Clin Orthop Relat Res 1993;220–2.
76. Mullins JF, Sallis JG. Recurrent sprain of the ankle joint with diastasis. J Bone Joint Surg Br 1958;40(2):270–3.
77. Castaing J, Le Chevallier PL, Meunier M. Repeated sprain or recurring subluxation of the tibio-tarsal joint. A simple technic of external ligamentoplasty. Rev Chir Orthop Reparatrice Appar Mot 1961;47:598–608 [in French].
78. Olerud C. The effect of the syndesmotic screw on the extension capacity of the ankle joint. Arch Orthop Trauma Surg 1985;104:299–302.
79. Tornetta P 3rd, Spoo JE, Reynolds FA, et al. Overtightening of the ankle syndesmosis: is it really possible? J Bone Joint Surg Am 2001;83:489–92.
80. Ebraheim NA, Mekhail AO, Gargasz SS. Ankle fractures involving the fibula proximal to the distal tibiofibular syndesmosis. Foot Ankle Int 1997;18:513–21.
81. Harper MC. The deltoid ligament. An evaluation of need for surgical repair. Clin Orthop Relat Res 1988;156–68.

82. Cox S, Mukherjee DP, Ogden AL, et al. Distal tibiofibular syndesmosis fixation: a cadaveric, simulated fracture stabilization study comparing bioabsorbable and metallic single screw fixation. J Foot Ankle Surg 2005;44:144–51.
83. Hovis WD, Kaiser BW, Watson JT, et al. Treatment of syndesmotic disruptions of the ankle with bioabsorbable screw fixation. J Bone Joint Surg Am 2002;84: 26–31.
84. Sinisaari IP, Luthje PM, Mikkonen RH. Ruptured tibio-fibular syndesmosis: comparison study of metallic to bioabsorbable fixation. Foot Ankle Int 2002;23: 744–8.
85. Thordarson DB, Samuelson M, Shepherd LE, et al. Bioabsorbable versus stainless steel screw fixation of the syndesmosis in pronation-lateral rotation ankle fractures: a prospective randomized trial. Foot Ankle Int 2001;22:335–8.
86. Bostman OM, Pihlajamaki HK, Partio EK, et al. Clinical biocompatibility and degradation of polylevolactide screws in the ankle. Clin Orthop Relat Res 1995;320:101–9.
87. Hovis WD, Bucholz RW. Polyglycolide bioabsorbable screws in the treatment of ankle fractures. Foot Ankle Int 1997;18:128–31.
88. Schafer D, Hintermann B. Arthroscopic assessment of the chronic unstable ankle joint. Knee Surg Sports Traumatol Arthrosc 1996;4:48–52.

Acute Lateral Ankle Ligament Ruptures in the Athlete
The Role of Surgery

Gino M.M.J. Kerkhoffs, MD, PhD*, C. Niek Van Dijk, MD, PhD

KEYWORDS

- Lateral ankle ligament rupture • Ankle ligament reconstruction • Foot inversion
- Athletes

KEY POINTS

- Greater ankle stability and an earlier return to sports can be achieved with early operative reconstruction following acute lateral ligament injury.
- The results of surgical reconstruction with single-surgeon series are superior to multi-surgeon series.
- Early surgical reconstruction should be considered in high-level sportsmen.

BACKGROUND

A great number of athletes suffer from a traumatic injury to the lateral ankle ligament. In fact, the magnitude of this "simple" injury is such that lateral ankle ligament injuries involve about 25% of all injuries of the locomotor system and account for up to 40% of all athletic injuries. Lateral ankle ligament injuries are most commonly seen in athletes participating in basketball, soccer, running, and ballet or dance.[1–5] Up to 53% of basketball injuries and 29% of soccer injuries can be attributed to ankle injuries, and 12% of time lost in football is due to ankle injuries.[1,2]

The most common mechanism of injury is internal rotation (inversion) of the plantar-flexed foot (toes on ground and heel up). Injury occurs to the anterior talofibular ligament first, followed to a varying degree by injury to the calcaneofibular ligament. The posterior talofibular ligament is usually uninjured unless there is a frank dislocation of the ankle. Together, these ligaments form the lateral ligament complex.

Optimal treatment for these injuries has been debated for many years. During the last decade, mainly functional treatment using a lace-up support in combination with exercise training was advocated, based on evidence from the available literature.[6,7] The aim of this article is to review the latest literature and propose an updated

Department of Orthopedic Surgery, Orthopedic Research Center Amsterdam, Academic Medical Center, Meibergdreef 9, Amsterdam 1105 AZ, The Netherlands
* Corresponding author.
E-mail address: g.m.kerkhoffs@amc.nl

Foot Ankle Clin N Am 18 (2013) 215–218
http://dx.doi.org/10.1016/j.fcl.2013.02.003
1083-7515/13/$ – see front matter Crown Copyright © 2013 Published by Elsevier Inc. All rights reserved.

evidence-based treatment regimen for acute lateral ankle ligament rupture in the athlete. It has been hypothesized that for athletes with such injuries, surgical treatment could be the preferred alternative to functional treatment.

TREATMENT OF LATERAL ANKLE LIGAMENT INJURIES IN THE ATHLETE

Although there has been much research conducted into lateral ankle ligament injury, there remains a lack of consensus as to the best treatment of such injuries, specifically in the athlete. The current best evidence for the treatment of acute lateral ankle ligament injuries in the general population was summarized in the recently published Dutch National Guideline,[8] and this was subsequently used by experts in the field for a debate on the best treatment for acute lateral ligament injuries in athletes. In the aforementioned guideline, the recommendations were set based on evidence from published scientific research. The quality of included articles was assessed by epidemiologists on the basis of "evidence-based guideline development" assessment forms (EBRO), and classified in order of probative and scientific value.[8]

A patient suffering from an acute lateral ankle ligament injury benefits from the use of so-called RICE (rest, ice [cryotherapy], compression, and elevation)[8–14]; also, the use of nonsteroidal anti-inflammatory drugs is recommended in the acute phase of recovery.[15,16] Manual mobilizations of the ankle must be discouraged.[17–19] Ultrasound therapy, laser therapy, and electrotherapy have no added value.[20–24] More than 2 weeks of immobilization in a lower leg cast is not an effective treatment strategy.[6] However, a short period of plaster immobilization or similar rigid support could well facilitate a rapid decrease of pain and swelling, and can thus be helpful in this phase of the treatment.[25] Thereafter a functional treatment is recommended and, as part of this functional approach, the use of an ankle support is advocated. An elastic bandage gives fewer complications than tape, but is associated with a delayed return to work and sports. It seems that overall, a lace-up brace or semirigid brace is preferable. In professional athletes the use of tape can be considered, although this requires careful application because the risk of complications such as skin problems is greater than when a brace or elastic bandage is used.[7] Exercise therapy should also be recognized as an essential element of the functional treatment of acute lateral ankle ligament injury, and this form of therapy can also be effectively performed at home.[8,17] In the general population, functional treatment is preferred over surgical therapy.[7] However, in professional athletes surgical treatment may be considered on an individual basis.[8]

TREATMENT OF LATERAL ANKLE LIGAMENT INJURIES IN THE ATHLETE: THE ROLE OF SURGERY

At present, most patients with acute lateral ankle ligament injury are treated nonoperatively and surgical repair is reserved for patients with chronic, symptomatic lateral ankle ligament laxity. Review of the evidence from recent literature on this topic, including a Cochrane systematic review on surgical treatment of acute lateral ankle ligament injuries along with a comprehensive examination of all randomized controlled clinical trials comparing surgery with conservative treatment of these injuries, shows no clear superiority of one treatment approach over the other.[26] Given the risk of operative complications, the stiffness of the ankle joint, and the higher costs associated with surgical treatment, the best available option for most patients would be functional treatment of acute injuries with close follow-up to identify patients with complaints of chronic lateral ankle ligament laxity.[26]

However, the majority (n = 15) of the trials in this review were conducted at least 20 years ago and reflect previous practice, including the use of prolonged cast immobilization postoperatively. Such postsurgical rehabilitation has been open to debate and change to earlier mobilization, and it is therefore questionable as to how much of the evidence from these trials is applicable to current care for athletes suffering an acute lateral ankle ligament injury.

An increasingly important aspect in the care of injured high-level athletes in general is the time to the next event and the presence of residual complaints. For lateral ankle ligament injuries in athletes, the modern postsurgical treatment protocols mean that the time to return to sport will be similar, with or without surgery. The rehabilitation regime after direct anatomic repair of the ruptured ligaments has altered from 6 weeks in a lower-leg cast to 1 week in a cast and 2 weeks in a walking boot, followed by an active exercise protocol and the use of an ankle support. Therefore, the choice is between a straightforward return to sport with functional treatment on the one hand, and return to sport with an objectively more stable ankle after surgical treatment on the other.[26] Objective instability, as defined by a positive talar tilt on stress radiographs or positive anterior drawer sign, was significantly less common in the surgical treatment group.[26] Because higher objective instability is a predictor of future ankle sprains, an acute lateral ligament reconstruction can be considered in high-demand athletes.

Experts agree that the outcome of surgical repair of acute lateral ligament injuries is more likely to be positive if performed by an experienced surgeon.[27] This interesting viewpoint is currently under investigation through analysis of the current literature, to assess whether outcomes indeed differ significantly when only the results of expert surgeons are compared with functional treatment with lace-up support and exercise training. Because elite athletes are likely to be operated on by an expert foot/ankle or sports surgeon, this aspect of the argument in favor of acute repair for selected high-demand athletes is strengthened.

In conclusion, given the summary of the literature and the evidence-based arguments, the authors advocate a personal treatment approach for the athlete with an acute lateral ankle ligament injury. A direct anatomic repair of the ruptured ligaments by an expert foot/ankle or sports surgeon may be considered, to develop a more stable ankle joint at follow-up without compromising or delaying return to participation in sport.

REFERENCES

1. McKay GD, Goldie PA, Payne WR, et al. Ankle injuries in basketball: injury rate and risk factors. Br J Sports Med 2001;35:103-8.
2. Ekstrand J. The incidence of ankle sprains in football. Foot Ankle 1990;11:41-4.
3. Lindenfeld TN, Schmitt DJ, Hendy MP, et al. Incidence of injury in indoor soccer. Am J Sports Med 1994;22:364-71.
4. Bahr R, Lian O, Bahr IA. A twofold reduction on the incidence of acute ankle sprains in volleyball after the introduction of an injury prevention program: a prospective cohort study. Scand J Med Sci Sports 1999;7:172-7.
5. Creagh U, Reilly T. Training and injuries amongst elite female orienteers. J Sports Med Phys Fitness 1998;38:75-9.
6. Kerkhoffs GM, Rowe BH, Assendelft WJ, et al. Immobilisation for acute ankle sprain. A systematic review [review]. Arch Orthop Trauma Surg 2001;121(8):462-71.
7. Kerkhoffs GM, Struijs PA, Marti RK, et al. Functional treatments for acute ruptures of the lateral ankle ligament: a systematic review [review]. Acta Orthop Scand 2003;74(1):69-77.
8. Kerkhoffs GM, van den Bekerom M, Elders LA, et al. Diagnosis, treatment and prevention of ankle sprains: an evidence-based clinical guideline. Br J Sports Med 2012;46(12):854-60.

9. Bleakley C, McDonough S, MacAuley D. The use of ice in the treatment of acute soft-tissue injury: a systematic review of randomized controlled trials. Am J Sports Med 2004;32(1):251–61.
10. Cote DJ, Prentice WE, Hooker DN, et al. Comparison of three treatment procedures for minimizing ankle sprain swelling. Phys Ther 1988;68:1064–76.
11. Airaksinen O, Kolari PJ, Miettienen H. Elastic bandages and intermittent pneumatic compression for treatment of acute ankle sprains. Arch Phys Med Rehabil 1990;71(6):380–3.
12. Rucinsky JJ, Hooker DN, Prentice WE, et al. The effects of intermittent compression on oedema in postacute ankle sprains. J Orthop Sports Phys Ther 1991; 14(2):65–9.
13. Tsang KK, Hertel J, Denegar CR. Volume decreases after elevation and intermittent compression of postacute ankle sprains are negated by gravity-dependent positioning. J Athl Train 2003;38(4):320–4.
14. Bleakley CM, McDonough SM, MacAuley DC, et al. Cryotherapy for acute ankle sprains: a randomised controlled study of two different icing protocols. Br J Sports Med 2006;40(8):700–5.
15. Almekinders LC. Anti-inflammatory treatment of muscular injuries in sport: an update of recent studies. Sports Med 1999;28:383–8.
16. van Dijk CN. CBO-guideline for diagnosis and treatment of the acute ankle injury. Ned Tijdschr Geneeskd 1999;143:2097–101.
17. Van der Wees PH, Lenssen AF, Hendriks HJ, et al. Effectiveness of exercise therapy and manual mobilisation in acute ankle sprain and functional instability: a systematic review. Aust J Physiother 2006;52:27–37.
18. Bleakley CM, McDonough SM, MacAuley DC. Some conservative strategies are effective when added to controlled mobilisation with external support after acute ankle sprain: a systematic review. Aust J Physiother 2008;54(1):7–20.
19. Brantingham JW, Globe G, Pollard H, et al. Manipulative therapy for lower extremity conditions: expansion of literature review. J Manipulative Physiol Ther 2009;32(1):53–71.
20. Barker AT, Barlow PS, Porter J, et al. A double-blind clinical trial of lower power pulsed shortwave therapy in the treatment of a soft tissue injury. Phys Ther 1985;71(12):500–4.
21. Michlovitz S, Smith W, Watkins M. Ice and high voltage pulsed stimulation in treatment of acute lateral ankle sprains. J Orthop Sports Phys Ther 1988;9:301–4.
22. Pasila M, Visuri T, Sundholm A. Pulsating shortwave diathermy: value in treatment of recent ankle and foot sprains. Arch Phys Med Rehabil 1978;59(8):383–6.
23. Pennington GM, Danley DL, Sumko MH, et al. Pulsed, non-thermal, high-frequency electromagnetic energy (DIAPULSE) in the treatment of grade I and grade II ankle sprains. Mil Med 1993;158(2):101–4.
24. Wilson DH. Treatment of soft-tissue injuries by pulsed electrical energy. Br Med J 1972;2:269–70.
25. Lamb SE, Marsh JL, Hutton JL, et al, Collaborative Ankle Support Trial (CAST Group). Mechanical supports for acute, severe ankle sprain: a pragmatic, multi-centre, randomised controlled trial. Lancet 2009;373(9663):575–81.
26. Kerkhoffs GM, Handoll HH, de Bie R, et al. Surgical versus conservative treatment for acute injuries of the lateral ligament complex of the ankle in adults. Cochrane Database Syst Rev 2007;(2):CD000380.
27. van Dijk CN. The athletes' ankle: lateral ligament injury. Consensus Meeting ESSKA-AFAS. Warsaw, 2011.

Lisfranc Injury in the Athlete
Evidence Supporting Management from Sprain to Fracture Dislocation

Kyriacos I. Eleftheriou, MD, FRCS(Tr & Orth)*,
Peter F. Rosenfeld, FRCS(Tr & Orth)

KEYWORDS

- Lisfranc • Foot • Injury • Athletes

KEY POINTS

- Lisfranc injuries are uncommon, but their prompt and accurate diagnosis in athletes is essential in preventing career-ending injury.
- Undisplaced injuries have an excellent result with nonoperative treatment.
- The presence of any displacement warrants open reduction and anatomic fixation. Current evidence mostly supports screw fixation. Plate fixation may, however, avoid joint intrusion and has merit.
- Athletes with significantly displaced injuries should be warned of the risk of a poor outcome. Recent evidence, however, suggests that return to elite competitive sports is still likely if patients are managed surgically.
- Severe injuries may have better outcomes with limited arthrodesis.

Injuries to the foot comprise approximately 16% of all sports-related injuries,[1] with midfoot sprains being the second most common athletic foot injury only after injuries to the metatarsophalangeal joint, occurring in 4% of American football players per year.[2] The Lisfranc joint is the articulation between the more rigid midfoot and the relatively flexible forefoot. The correct identification and management of disruption of this articulation is essential in optimizing the outcome of these potentially career-ending injuries in athletes.

The rigid midfoot acts as a strong lever arm during gait. It is made of a complex bony anatomy of the metatarsal, the cuneiforms, and the cuboid bones, supported by transverse, longitudinal, and oblique ligaments. The transverse ligaments are absent between the bases of the first and second metatarsals, producing a "weak" area which, with injury, may lead to the Lisfranc injury.

The authors have nothing to disclose.
Department of Trauma and Orthopaedics, St Mary's Hospital, Praed Street, London W2 1NY, UK
* Corresponding author.
E-mail address: akis22@gmail.com

ANATOMY

The osseous geometry between the 3 cuneiforms and cuboid proximally and the 5 metatarsals distally as well as the capsuloligamentous structures are essential to the critical stability of the Lisfranc articulation and the maintenance of both the transverse and longitudinal arch of the foot.

The base of the second metatarsal is the "keystone" recessed in a mortise between the medial and lateral cuneiforms, which provides direct osseous stability to the articulation, with a shallow mortise being a positive risk factor for a Lisfranc injury.[3] The strong capsuloligamentous structures provide indirect stability.[3] Plantar and dorsal ligaments span the articulation in longitudinal and oblique directions between the tarsal and metatarsal bones while transverse ligaments interconnect the metatarsal bases. The plantar ligaments are stronger, which may explain the dorsal direction of dislocations.

Whereas the presence of strong interosseous ligaments provides significant stability to the articulation, these are absent between the medial and middle cuneiforms and the bases of the first and second metatarsal. The Lisfranc ligament is located plantarly between the medial cuneiform and the base of the second metatarsal. It is the largest (~1 cm in length and 0.5 cm in width) and strongest of the interosseous ligaments and is regarded as essential for the overall stability of the articulation (**Fig. 1**). The dorsal ligaments have only one-third of the strength of the Lisfranc ligament and are also weaker than the remaining plantar ligaments.[4–6] Sequential sectioning of the relevant ligaments has shown that both the Lisfranc ligament and the plantar ligament between the second and third metatarsals need to be divided before transverse instability is observed, and longitudinal instability is produced by sectioning of the interosseous ligament between the medial and middle cuneiforms.[7,8]

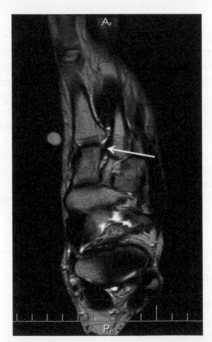

Fig. 1. Magnetic resonance image showing Lisfranc ligament (*arrow*).

It is also important to be aware of structures adjacent to the articulation that may be involved in injury. These structures include the perforating branch of the dorsalis pedis artery passing plantarly through the first web space and the deep peroneal nerve. The tibialis anterior tendon, with its insertion over the dorsomedial aspect of the medial cuneiform and the base of the first metatarsal, may also impede reduction of the joint when entrapped after injury.[9,10]

The midfoot is usually described as 3 columns. The medial column consists of the navicular, medial cuneiform and the first metatarsal. Whereas coronal motion in the medial column is minimal, there is some movement in the frontal and sagittal planes (3°–4°) with dorsiflexion linked with inversion and plantarflexion with eversion.[9] The lateral column is the most mobile with up to 10° movement in both the coronal and sagittal planes, and consists of the cuboid and the fourth and fifth metatarsals. Its increased mobility would help explain why instability after injury is better tolerated, and development of symptomatic lateral column arthritis is rare.[9] The middle column is the most rigid articulation between the second and third metatarsals and the middle and lateral cuneiforms. It provides an effective lever arm during gait and experiences the largest forces during the heel-rise phase of gait.[11]

EPIDEMIOLOGY AND MECHANISMS OF INJURY

Lisfranc injuries are uncommon. An incidence rate of 1 in 55,000 people has been reported for the United States annually, accounting for only 0.2% of all fractures.[12,13] However, this may be an underestimate, as up to one-third may be missed on initial presentation.[14–17] Males are 2 to 4 times more likely to sustain an injury, likely because of their higher participation in activities involving high-speed injuries.[18] Injuries to the articulation may be due to indirect forces (bending and twisting moments applied to the midfoot) or direct forces such as crush injuries. In view of the lack of a ligamentous connection between the first and second metatarsal bases, the keystone arrangement of the second metatarsal between the surrounding cuneiforms is essential for stability. When a sufficient force is applied with the foot in significant hyperplantarflexion, however, the second metatarsal is at risk of dislocating dorsally, with little support provided from the dorsal ligaments. When this occurs, both the bony keystone congruity and the strength of the Lisfranc ligament often lead to a fracture of the base of the second metatarsal that is seen on plain radiographs and has been termed the fleck sign (**Fig. 2**). In high-energy injuries, as usually seen in motor vehicle accidents, the foot is pushed into hyperplantarflexion with a valgus or varus component as it is planted on the floor or brake pedal after impact. The large energy disrupts the Lisfranc articulation and is usually associated with significant instability as well as the potential for neurovascular injury and compartment syndrome.[19]

Injury in the Athlete

While high-energy injuries such as motor vehicle accidents are more common than low-energy injuries such as a fall from height (58% vs 42%, respectively[20]), midfoot sprains occurring after an indirect low-energy force are much more common in the athletic population, and present in a more subtle manner. Midfoot sprains are the second most common athletic foot injury (after injuries to the metatarsophalangeal joint) and occur in 4% of football players per year,[2] with offensive linemen being the commonest players to sustain the injury (29.2%).[2]

Two main mechanisms of injury have been described in athletes. The first occurs in athletes that have their foot in a strap, such as equestrians and windsurfers, and is the classic mechanism often mentioned of soldiers on horseback falling off with their foot

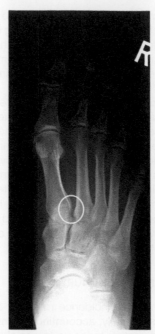

Fig. 2. Avulsion of the base (*circled*) of the second metatarsal, pathognomonic of a Lisfranc injury (the fleck sign), can be subtle.

trapped in the stirrups, thus sustaining a hyperplantarflexion force while the body falls backward. The second is often seen in American football players, when their foot is plantarflexed with the metatarsophalangeal joints maximally dorsiflexed, thus sustaining a direct force onto their heel by a falling player that leads to hyperplantar-flexion.[21] Other mechanisms described involve hyperplantarflexion of the foot when baseball players slide onto a fixed base, or parachutists land on a fully plantarflexed foot.[19] Injuries have been described in other sporting disciplines such as soccer, basketball, and running, but also appear to have a high incidence in gymnastics, which may be due to direct forces that occur when the foot hits the balance beam.[22] Equestrian sports also see a high incidence of such injuries, either when the foot is stuck in the stirrup with the rider falling, or when the foot is caught between horse and ground.[23] Although such injuries have been described in ballet they are much rarer in comparison with other disciplines, which may be due to a combination of the stability of the pointe shoe, the physiologic control of the dancer, and possibly a degree of increased stability of the joint during the en-pointe position, as suggested by a biomechanical study.[24]

CLASSIFICATIONS

The original classification of Lisfranc injuries was described by Quenu and Kuss in 1909, based on their column concept that divided injuries into homolateral, isolated, and divergent.[20] This classification has since been modified by Hardcastle and colleagues,[25] then by Myerson and colleagues.[14] The latter is the most common classification system used, and is divided into 3 categories (**Fig. 3**): Type A (Total Incongruity) involves complete displacement of all the metatarsal in either a medial or

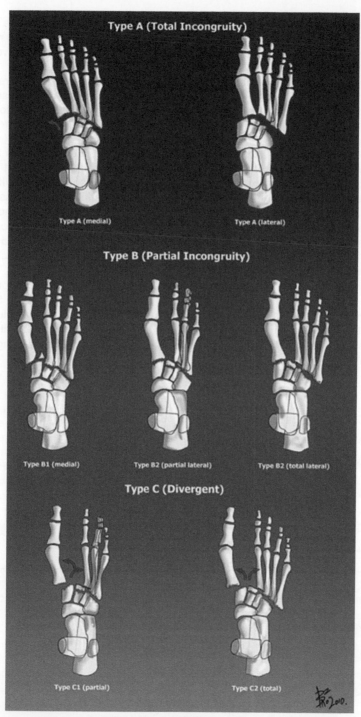

Fig. 3. Myerson classifications of Lisfranc injuries. (*From* Stavlas P, Roberts CS, Xypnitos FN, et al. The role of reduction and internal fixation of Lisfranc fracture-dislocations: a systematic review of the literature. Int Orthop 2012;34:1083–91; with permission from Springer Science and Business Media.)

lateral pattern; Type B (Partial Incongruity) involves displacement of 1 or more (but not all) metatarsals and may be medial (B1) or lateral (B2/B3); Type C (Divergent) refers to injuries when all (total C2) or some (partial C1) of the metatarsals are divergently displaced (see **Fig. 3**).

Low-energy injuries, such as those seen in the athletic population, are more subtle. Nunley and Vertullo[26] thus put forward a classification system that addresses such injuries, based on clinical examination, comparative weight-bearing radiographs, and bone scans. In Stage I injuries they included patients who are not able to participate in sport and have pain in the Lisfranc region, but whose plain weight-bearing radiographs show no displacement; bone scans, however, are positive. In Stage II injuries there is a diastasis of 1 to 5 mm on the anteroposterior (AP) weight-bearing plain radiograph with no loss of midfoot arch on the lateral radiograph. Stage III injuries show a diastasis of greater than 5 mm on the AP weight-bearing film, with loss of midfoot arch and height and a reduced distance between the fifth metatarsal and medial cuneiform on the lateral radiograph.[26] These investigators recommended nonoperative treatment for stage I injuries (undisplaced), and anatomic reduction and fixation for Stage II (diastasis with no arch height loss) and Stage III (diastasis with arch height loss) injuries.

It is important at this point to note the discrepancy between the descriptive and figurative (**Fig. 4**) classification as described by Nunley and Vertullo[26]: Stage II injuries were classified as those with a diastasis of 1 to 5 mm while their illustrative classification (see **Fig. 4**) showed this as diastasis of 2 to 5 mm; Stage III injuries were illustrated as again having a diastasis of 2 to 5 mm with loss of longitudinal arch height.

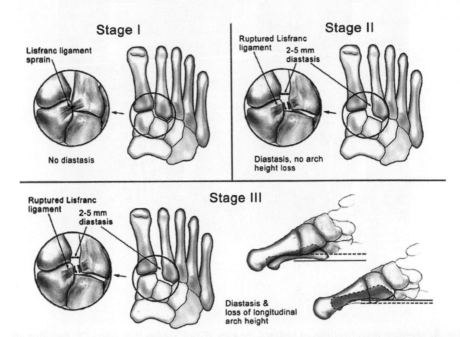

Fig. 4. Midfoot sprain classification system as described by Nunley and Vertullo. (*From* Nunley JA, Vertullo CJ. Classification, investigation, and management of midfoot sprains: Lisfranc injuries in the athlete. Am J Sports Med 2002;30:871; with permission.)

PRESENTATION AND EXAMINATION FINDINGS

Although Lisfranc injuries from high-energy mechanisms present with more prominent examination findings such as significant bruising, swelling, pain, and instability, a proportion is still missed. In the low-energy injuries for which the index of suspicion may be lower and the signs more subtle, they may be even more difficult to detect. This situation is not made easier by the athletes themselves, who often underestimate the injury and try to walk it off.

The history of the mechanism of injury provides important clues. Pain, swelling, and tenderness in the midfoot should raise suspicion, while pain on passive pronation and supination of the forefoot at the tarsometatarsal (TMT) joints may produce significant pain and show evidence of instability. Passive dorsiflexion and abduction of the forefoot may also produce pain, while dorsal bruising over the forefoot may be a late sign.[19] Assessment for associated injuries including local neurovascular injury is also important, as well as comparison with the contralateral foot. Bilateral injuries may, however, be seen in windsurfers and parachutists.[19]

IMAGING

Anteroposterior, 30° oblique, and lateral radiographs should be the first examinations requested. Weight-bearing views (an ankle block may be considered to allow this) and comparison views with the contralateral uninjured foot may be helpful (**Fig. 5**). Radiographic findings consistent with a Lisfranc injury are detailed in **Box 1**.

If weight-bearing views are not possible, one should consider stress views usually obtained under anesthesia. To perform these, one has to stabilize the hindfoot and apply a supination and abduction/adduction stress to the forefoot. Although displacement of more than 2 mm is often taken to be suggestive of instability, cadaveric studies have shown that a diastasis of 1.3 mm may be significant in differentiating between the intact and torn Lisfranc ligament[32] while plain radiographs may not reliably pick up malalignment of 1 to 2 mm.[33]

Computed tomography (CT) scanning, especially with multiplanar reconstructions, provides a more accurate assessment of minor displacement, showing occult fractures and helping with preoperative planning.[34–37] Nevertheless, it is a non–weight-bearing investigation and in undisplaced injuries may be of little benefit.[9] Magnetic resonance imaging (MRI) scans, on the other hand, may be superior in identifying

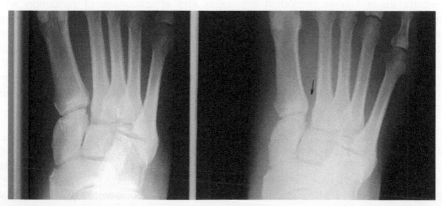

Fig. 5. Weight-bearing views are important to demonstrate the diastasis (*arrow*) between the first and second metatarsals.

Box 1
Radiographic findings consistent with Lisfranc injuries

Loss of alignment of medial border of second metatarsal with medial border of medial cuneiform[27]

Diastasis greater than 2 mm between base of first and second metatarsals on the AP view,[28] or a difference greater than 1 mm than that of the uninjured contralateral foot (see **Fig. 5**)[29]

Loss of alignment between the medial border of the fourth metatarsal and medial border of cuboid on oblique view[28,30]

Presence of the fleck sign on the AP view representing an avulsion of the Lisfranc ligament (see **Fig. 2**)[28]

Loss of alignment between the plantar aspect of the fifth metatarsal and medial cuneiform on the lateral view[29,31]

Stage I injuries whereby bone marrow edema around the Lisfranc joint or injury to the Lisfranc ligament are better depicted, and the absence of such findings may make further investigations unnecessary.[35,38–40] Disruption of the plantar ligament between the first cuneiform and the bases of the second and third metatarsals on MRI has been shown to be the strongest predictor of intraoperative instability, with sensitivity and predictive values of 94%.[41]

As previously described, bone-scan findings were used as part of the classification system of Nunley and Vertullo to identify Stage I injuries.[26] Based on the evidence discussed here, the authors sequentially proceed with weight-bearing views, CT, and/or MRI scans to define the level of injury and thus optimize treatment for the injured athlete, as discussed later.

MANAGEMENT

Posttraumatic arthritis is the commonest complication after Lisfranc injuries, and ranges from mild degenerative changes to complete loss of joint space seen in almost half of patients.[20] Although the importance of anatomic reduction in optimizing outcome has always been highlighted,[36,42] the rarity and varied presentation of such injuries make it difficult to study and there is, therefore, a lack of well-designed randomized controlled studies. More information is needed to decide on the optimum treatment for these injuries, including the value and effectiveness of reduction and fixation, the type of fixation, and the relative benefits of alternative management such as primary or delayed arthrodesis. Nevertheless, most investigators believe that the development of degenerative changes is higher when the injury and its extent has been unrecognized or partially treated, when the anatomy has not been restored, and when the injury is purely ligamentous.[20] A delay of operative treatment of more than 6 months as well as a concomitant compensation claim are associated with a poorer outcome.[43]

Nonoperative Management

Although a plaster cast may initially hold an anatomic closed reduction, as the swelling subsides this is often lost.[14] Nonoperative treatment should be reserved for athletes with stable Stage I (Nunley and Vertullo) injuries, and good results have been reported whether the athletes are kept in a non–weight-bearing cast for 6 weeks (93% excellent results)[26] or allowed immediate weight bearing in an orthotic.[2] Others, including the authors, recommend an initial protective period of 2 weeks in a non–weight-bearing cast or boot, before patients are reexamined; absence of both tenderness and diastasis on repeat weight-bearing radiographs confirm stability, and a return to activities is allowed as tolerated, perhaps with a further period of protection weight bearing as tolerated in a long walker-boot with orthotic support.[19] Persistence of tenderness requires further immobilization. Some investigators suggest the use of a well-molded arch support orthotic for athletic activities for 3 to 4 months after this time.[19]

Despite the variation in nonoperative treatment for Stage I injuries, the evidence shows that athletes with such injuries will recover and are usually able to return to sport.[2,21,26] Patients with diastasis of more than 2 mm treated conservatively had worse results or had a prolonged recovery.[2,21,26] Such poor results of nonoperative treatment in the presence of instability or displacement have been reported by others in both the athletic[44,45] and nonathletic populations.[14,46–48] As previously mentioned, however, a diastasis of less than 2 mm can still be significant and consistent with a complete tear of the Lisfranc ligament[32]; the authors, therefore, believe that such injuries should still be operatively treated if identified, especially in the elite athlete.

Operative Management

Although there is consensus that any unstable injury (ie, greater than Stage I) should undergo operative treatment, there is still controversy with regard to its timing, the type of fixation, the postoperative management, the need for removal of metalwork, and whether a primary or delayed arthrodesis would provide optimum treatment. Most evidence does stem from traumatic nonathletic injuries, although limited evidence from studies in the athletic population is now available to help guide treatment.[2,21,22,26,49] These issues are discussed here.

Reduction and fixation

Closed reduction may be possible, although some argue that restoring congruency of the articulation is best achieved by open reduction.[50] Open reduction can be achieved by traction with finger traps and applying plantarflexion and supination of the forefoot, followed by dorsiflexion and pronation.[51] Percutaneous fixation may then be used, but if one is unable to reduce the displacement in a closed manner, open reduction and internal fixation should be undertaken.

Although K-wire pinning has been described for definitive fixation in partial incongruity injuries,[17,52,53] screw fixation is recommended, and is supported by biomechanical evidence that demonstrates greater stability of the medial and middle columns,[54] which can allow gentle compression of the joint (**Fig. 6**).[46,50] It also avoids redisplacement and redislocation with premature removal of the pins, as well as issues with pin-tract infection and migration.[14,50] Literature shows that screw fixation is preferred (82.8%) after open reduction (73.7%), usually with 3.5- or 4.0-mm screws.[20]

Operative reduction and fixation of the medial and middle columns should be undertaken first, but the order and exact stabilization of the joints does vary in the literature and will depend on preoperative and intraoperative findings. The goal is to reduce and stabilize the joints appropriately, and generally the second TMT joint, as the keystone, should be stabilized first, followed by reconstruction of the medial cuneiform–second metatarsal articulation. The neighboring first and third TMT joints are assessed for stability and stabilized as necessary. K-wires may be used to stabilize the fourth and fifth TMT articulations if necessary. Assessment of the intercuneiform joint stability at the end of the procedure is also essential, and any instability is also addressed (**Fig. 7**). Other surgeons, however, start with fixation from the medial cuneiform to the base of the second metatarsal and from the medial cuneiform to the intermediate

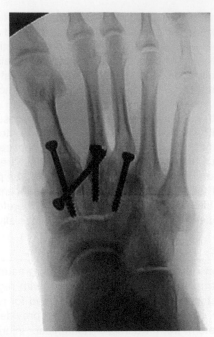

Fig. 6. Screw fixation for a Lisfranc injury.

cuneiform for Myerson B1 injuries, and from the medial cuneiform to the second meta-tarsal base for B2 injuries.[9] Most surgeons appear to only stabilize the lateral column if still unstable,[17,47,48,52] and do so using K-wires (rather than screw fixation[50]), taking into consideration the relative greater motion and the rare occurrence of posttraumatic osteoarthritis in the lateral column.

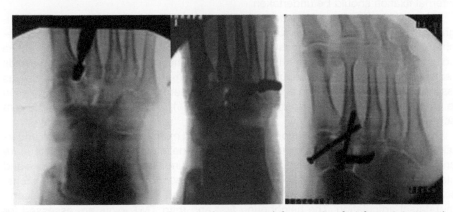

Fig. 7. Intraoperative imaging of the technique used for repair of Lisfranc injuries. The second tarsometatarsal (TMT) joint is anatomically reduced and fixed first; the other joints can then be reduced around this. The medial cuneiform-second metatarsal articulation is then stabilized, before the first and third TMT joints are assessed and fixed as necessary, followed by the fourth and fifth TMT articulations. Intercuneiform joint stability at the end of the procedure is also essential, and any instability is addressed.

Plate fixation
With the availability of strong new implants, an extra-articular approach to fixation should be considered to avoid damage to the articular surfaces of the joints, especially when one considers that a 3.5-mm screw can damage 2% to 4.8% of the TMT joint's articular cartilage (this cadaveric evidence may indeed be an underestimate when one considers the additional thermal damage in vivo).[55] Biomechanical models have shown dorsal plating to provide a construct at least as stable as transarticular screws,[55,56] with plantar plating providing even more stability (**Fig. 8**).[56,57] Locking plates also appear to provide stronger fixation than nonlocking plates.[58] Although the initial concerns of issues with soft-tissue irritation have been addressed with new low-profile designs, there is no strong clinical evidence to suggest their use at the moment. The authors use locking plates primarily, to avoid compromising the joint, and do not routinely remove them.

Other implants for fixation
In an attempt to avoid both the need of screw removal and leaving the screws in situ, some surgeons have used bioabsorbable screws (eg, polylactide screws).[9] Studies of their use in other skeletal areas showed acceptable stiffness,[59] and one clinical study showed that their use in management of Lisfranc injuries was safe and without reaction.[60] Issues with loss of fixation and joint damage with degradation of these screws are still of concern, however.[55]

The trend to provide a more physiologic fixation to the Lisfranc articulation and to reduce the need for screw removal has led some surgeons to use a suture-button fixation (Tightrope; Arthrex, Naples, FL).[61] In a cadaveric biomechanical model, the separation between the first metatarsal at the metaphyseal flare and the perpendicular corresponding point on the base of the second metatarsal was measured; less

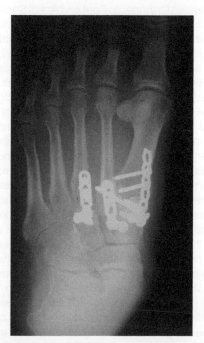

Fig. 8. Extra-articular plating used to stabilize the midfoot.

diastasis was observed using a 4.0-mm cannulated screw compared with a suture-button fixation, so the authors do not recommend the use of the latter at the moment.[62]

Surgical Approaches

Several surgical approaches have been described, including a variation of 2 or 3 dorsal longitudinal incisions to allow access to the 3 columns[9,18,50] or a transverse incision.[63,64] The use of the latter may be advantageous with regard to access, but the disruption of the cutaneous blood supply is of concern. A modification of the transverse incision in a zone proximal to the arcuate artery and distal to the lateral tarsal artery has been described, with some evidence that it may not increase wound complications.[63] Arthroscopic reduction has also been described.[65]

Arthrodesis

Primary arthrodesis has been advocated for complex injuries by some investigators.[66] It is argued that when there are 2 large fragments at the base of the second metatarsal, with the Lisfranc ligament being attached to 1 of the fragments, fixation may provide stability. However, in the presence of more comminution it is unlikely that fixation will reconstruct the joint without subsequent arthritic degeneration, and fusion is no more difficult than fixation.[66] What has also been of interest recently is the possibility that purely ligamentous injuries may fare better with primary arthrodesis, as such injuries are less likely to stabilize following fixation and may go on to develop degenerative changes.[46] In a randomized controlled trial of 41 patients with isolated acute or subacute injuries and a mean follow-up of 42.5 months, the patients who were managed with arthrodesis were able to reach 92% of their subjective preinjury level of physical or sports activity, compared with only 65% of those who had open reduction and fixation (ORIF).[47] What was not clear in the study, however, was the preinjury level of activity (and therefore athletic involvement) of such patients. The patients who underwent ORIF also had worse American Orthopedic Foot and Ankle Society Midfoot Scale Score outcomes, and a significant proportion (15 of 20) had loss of correction and degenerative changes, ranging from minor loss of correction to significant collapse and degenerative changes.[47] The investigators postulated that soft-tissue healing was inadequate to support reduction in such injuries despite fixation. Furthermore, patients in both groups had sustained both low-energy and high-energy injuries. These findings cannot, therefore, be easily extrapolated to guide management for a highly athletic population.

In another study, Mulier and colleagues[67] compared ORIF of severe Lisfranc injuries (16 patients) with partial (5 patients) and complete (6 patients; including the lateral column) arthrodesis. At the 30-month follow-up, patients who underwent complete fusion had more pain than the ORIF and partial arthrodesis groups (which had a similar level of pain) as assessed by the Baltimore Painful Foot Score; in addition, the former exhibited a higher proportion of forefoot stiffness, loss of metatarsal arch, and sympathetic dystrophy compared with the other groups. Complete fusion gave worse results (likely due to the stiffness of the relatively mobile lateral column). Although the functional scores were similar to the group that underwent ORIF and partial arthrodesis, 94% of the ORIF group had developed degenerative changes on plain radiographs. It was thus argued that, because a significant proportion of these patients with radiographic degenerative changes will require fusion anyway, a partial arthrodesis may be the preferred option,[66] and professional athletes have been reported to be able to return to high-level sport after Lisfranc fusions.[68] Based on these findings, the authors believe that primary partial arthrodesis should be considered in patients with either comminution or significantly displaced purely ligamentous injury, as this may also obviate metalwork removal at a later stage after fixation.

Although secondary corrective arthrodesis is a useful salvage procedure, and can significantly reduce pain and improve function in patients with missed Lisfranc fracture dislocations or in patients with secondary degenerative changes,[69–72] it should not serve as an alternative to primary ORIF, which leads to better overall results in both pain and function.[17]

Timing of surgery

There is little evidence to allow recommendation on the best timing for surgery. Although significantly poorer results are seen if operative treatment is delayed for more than 6 months,[43] most surgeons would allow significant soft-tissue swelling to settle down, and a 1- to 2-week delay has not been shown to negatively affect outcomes of ORIF.[9,46,73] Compartment syndrome is uncommon in sports-related Lisfranc injuries but, if suspected, prompt fasciotomies may be required.[9]

Postoperative protocol and removal of screws

Most surgeons agree on postoperative protection after fixation for at least 6 weeks,[20] but this may be extended depending on the degree of injury. Although K-wires are usually removed before weight bearing to avoid their breakage, the routine removal of screws is not followed by all surgeons. Problems with screws are common after fixation, and require removal in approximately 16% of patients.[20] Some surgeons remove the screws only when patients are symptomatic,[46,47,74] so as to minimize common risks of repeat surgery such as infection and neurovascular damage. Although some have reported no secondary displacement when screws are routinely removed at 8 weeks after surgery,[17] loss of reduction has been seen even following removal at 3 months.[47]

COMPLICATIONS AND PROGNOSIS

Short-term complications include compartment syndrome, neurovascular injury, wound problems, and deep vein thrombosis. Certainly metalwork problems are very common in the long term, leading to requirement for removal in 16% of patients, as well as the development of arthritis of the midfoot, instability, and flat-foot deformity.[51] Although radiographic degenerative changes may be seen in almost half of patients with Lisfranc injuries,[20] not all will be symptomatic and there is a lack of association between the extent of arthritis and symptoms.

Athletes with Stage I and Stage II injuries have been reported to be able to return to sport activity as early as 12 to 14 weeks, with no evidence that operative treatment may expedite this time.[2,21,26] The current evidence is limited to providing more accurate information on prognosis of more complex injuries in the athletic population; fortunately, sports-related injuries are usually low-energy with a low incidence of Stage III injuries (or greater), which have a worse outcome and will be unlikely to achieve the greater than 90% excellent results of Stage I and II injuries.[26] Although a low rate of return to elite competition has been reported in female gymnasts,[22] in a recent study of 15 elite soccer and rugby players surgically treated for ligamentous (8 athletes) and bony (7 athletes) Lisfranc injuries, only 1 athlete with a ligamentous injury retired. The others returned to training at a mean time of 20.2 weeks and to full competition at 25.6 weeks. Patients with purely ligamentous injuries returned to training slightly earlier. All patients were surgically treated by screw fixation between the medial cuneiform and base of the second metatarsal, with dorsal bridge-plating across any unstable TMT joints of the medial or middle columns. All metalwork was removed at 12 to 16 weeks unless a fusion procedure was performed.[49]

THE AUTHORS' ALGORITHM

What appears to be clear is that Stage I injuries as defined by Nunley and Vertullo[26] have excellent results with nonoperative treatment. The evidence provided here suggests that injuries with greater than 2 mm diastasis benefit from ORIF, which can provide excellent results and return to sport. Athletes with Stage III (or greater) injuries require anatomic reduction and fixation, but should be warned of the unfavorable outcomes of such injuries.

Looking at the evidence closely, however, the least clarity relates to Stage II (Nunley and Vertullo) injuries. Although their descriptive classification of a Stage II injury specified a diastasis of at least 1 mm,[26] both their illustrative classification (see **Fig. 4**) and the way results have been reported in other studies[2,21,26] use the 2-mm threshold as significant, and is used to differentiate Stage II from undisplaced injuries. Therefore, this leaves an unclassified subgroup of patients with 0 to 2 mm of displacement, this being the group that more often includes athletes. The management of this subgroup of minimally displaced Lisfranc injuries (ie, <2 mm) and their optimum management is still not clearly defined. Of note, again, is that cadaveric studies have shown that a diastasis of 1.3 mm may be significant in differentiating between

Table 1		
The authors' algorithm for the management of Lisfranc injuries in athletes		
Grade	Clinical and Imaging Findings	Management
1	Tender Lisfranc region on examination No displacement on plain weight-bearing (WB) radiographs No diastasis on CT Positive MRI scan	Initial protective period of 2 wk in a non–weight-bearing (NWB) cast or boot, before patients are reexamined Absence of tenderness and any diastasis on repeat WB radiographs would confirm stability. Protection in a WB boot with orthotic support for 4 wk and continued support in shoes for 3 mo. Return to activities after 6 wk as tolerated
2	≤2 mm displacement on WB anteroposterior (AP) radiographs (WB radiograph at 2 wk if unable to do initially in view of pain) AND/OR Diastasis on CT and/or intraoperative stress views in theater	Open reduction and internal fixation to ensure anatomic reduction Use of dorsal locking plate for medial and middle columns (remove only if symptomatic after 3 mo). Use of K-wires for lateral column if displaced (remove K-wires at 6 wk) NWB cast for 6 wk. WB removable boot for 6 wk NWB rehabilitation at 6 wk (swimming, water running, cycling) WB rehabilitation at 12 wk
3	>2 mm displacement on WB AP radiograph or Myerson Classification type injury	Open anatomic reduction and internal fixation. Stabilization or limited fusion (second tarsometatarsal joint primarily) for severe injuries. NWB cast for 6 wk NWB cast for 6 wk WB removable boot for 6 wk NWB rehabilitation at 6 wk (swimming, water running, cycling). WB rehabilitation at 12 wk Return to training at 16 wk if possible

the intact and torn Lisfranc ligament[32] while plain radiographs may not reliably pick up malalignment of 1 to 2 mm.[33]

The relative lack of good evidence in the exact management of such injuries makes a clear evidence-based approach to managing Lisfranc injuries difficult. In addition, there are few good data to support the possible advantages of the recent development of improved and stronger implants in providing stability to the TMT joint. Primary arthrodesis in unstable purely ligamentous injury may have advantages over fixation, but this has not been shown in the high-demand athletic population. Taking this into consideration, as well as the limited available evidence, the authors use a simple algorithm in managing Lisfranc injuries in their sporting patients (**Table 1**).

SUMMARY

Prompt and accurate diagnosis of Lisfranc injuries in athletes is essential in optimizing the result. Although the evidence is limited, undisplaced injuries should have an excellent result with nonoperative treatment. The presence of any displacement warrants open reduction and anatomic fixation. Most evidence supports screw fixation, but plate fixation avoids joint intrusion and is at least theoretically advantageous. It is imperative to warn athletes with significantly displaced injuries of a possible poor outcome and that this is a career-threatening injury, although some recent evidence suggests that return to elite competitive sports is still possible for most surgically managed injuries. Severe injuries can have better outcomes with limited arthrodesis.

REFERENCES

1. Garrick JG, Requa RK. The epidemiology of foot and ankle injuries in sports. Clin Sports Med 1988;7:29–36.
2. Meyer SA, Callaghan JJ, Albright JP, et al. Midfoot sprains in collegiate football players. Am J Sports Med 1994;22:392–401.
3. Peicha G, Labovitz J, Seibert FJ, et al. The anatomy of the joint as a risk factor for Lisfranc dislocation and fracture-dislocation. An anatomical and radiological case control study. J Bone Joint Surg Br 2002;84:981–5.
4. de Palma L, Santucci A, Sabetta SP, et al. Anatomy of the Lisfranc joint complex. Foot Ankle Int 1997;18:356–64.
5. Milankov M, Miljkovic N, Popovic N. Concomitant plantar tarsometatarsal (Lisfranc) and metatarsophalangeal joint dislocations. Arch Orthop Trauma Surg 2003;123:95–7.
6. Solan MC, Moorman CT 3rd, Miyamoto RG, et al. Ligamentous restraints of the second tarsometatarsal joint: a biomechanical evaluation. Foot Ankle Int 2001; 22:637–41.
7. Kaar S, Femino J, Morag Y. Lisfranc joint displacement following sequential ligament sectioning. J Bone Joint Surg Am 2007;89:2225–32.
8. Pearce CJ, Calder JD. Surgical anatomy of the midfoot. Knee Surg Sports Traumatol Arthrosc 2010;18:581–6.
9. DeOrio M, Erickson M, Usuelli FG, et al. Lisfranc injuries in sport. Foot Ankle Clin 2009;14:169–86.
10. DeBenedetti MJ, Evanski PM, Waugh TR. The unreducible Lisfranc fracture. Case report and literature review. Clin Orthop Relat Res 1978;238–40.
11. Root MI. Biomechanical examination of the foot. J Am Podiatry Assoc 1973;63: 28–9.
12. Aitken AP, Poulson D. Dislocations of the tarsometatarsal joint. J Bone Joint Surg Am 1963;45:246–60.

13. English TA. Dislocations of the metatarsal bone and adjacent toe. J Bone Joint Surg Br 1964;46:700–4.
14. Myerson MS, Fisher RT, Burgess AR, et al. Fracture dislocations of the tarsometatarsal joints: end results correlated with pathology and treatment. Foot Ankle 1986;6:225–42.
15. Perron AD, Brady WJ, Keats TE. Orthopedic pitfalls in the ED: Lisfranc fracture-dislocation. Am J Emerg Med 2001;19:71–5.
16. Philbin T, Rosenberg G, Sferra JJ. Complications of missed or untreated Lisfranc injuries. Foot Ankle Clin 2003;8:61–71.
17. Rammelt S, Schneiders W, Schikore H, et al. Primary open reduction and fixation compared with delayed corrective arthrodesis in the treatment of tarsometatarsal (Lisfranc) fracture dislocation. J Bone Joint Surg Br 2008;90:1499–506.
18. Desmond EA, Chou LB. Current concepts review: Lisfranc injuries. Foot Ankle Int 2006;27:653–60.
19. Lattermann C, Goldstein JL, Wukich DK, et al. Practical management of Lisfranc injuries in athletes. Clin J Sport Med 2007;17:311–5.
20. Stavlas P, Roberts CS, Xypnitos FN, et al. The role of reduction and internal fixation of Lisfranc fracture-dislocations: a systematic review of the literature. Int Orthop 2010;34:1083–91.
21. Shapiro MS, Wascher DC, Finerman GA. Rupture of Lisfranc's ligament in athletes. Am J Sports Med 1994;22:687–91.
22. Chilvers M, Donahue M, Nassar L, et al. Foot and ankle injuries in elite female gymnasts. Foot Ankle Int 2007;28:214–8.
23. Ceroni D, De Rosa V, De Coulon G, et al. The importance of proper shoe gear and safety stirrups in the prevention of equestrian foot injuries. J Foot Ankle Surg 2007;46:32–9.
24. Kadel N, Boenisch M, Teitz C, et al. Stability of Lisfranc joints in ballet pointe position. Foot Ankle Int 2005;26:394–400.
25. Hardcastle PH, Reschauer R, Kutscha-Lissberg E, et al. Injuries to the tarsometatarsal joint. Incidence, classification and treatment. J Bone Joint Surg Br 1982;64:349–56.
26. Nunley JA, Vertullo CJ. Classification, investigation, and management of midfoot sprains: Lisfranc injuries in the athlete. Am J Sports Med 2002;30:871–8.
27. Foster SC, Foster RR. Lisfranc's tarsometatarsal fracture-dislocation. Radiology 1976;120:79–83.
28. Tadros AM, Al-Hussona M. Bilateral tarsometatarsal fracture-dislocations: a missed work-related injury. Singapore Med J 2008;49:e234–5.
29. Faciszewski T, Burks RT, Manaster BJ. Subtle injuries of the Lisfranc joint. J Bone Joint Surg Am 1990;72:1519–22.
30. Sharma D, Khan F. Lisfranc fracture dislocations—an important and easily missed fracture in the emergency department. J R Army Med Corps 2002;148:44–7.
31. Stein RE. Radiological aspects of the tarsometatarsal joints. Foot Ankle 1983;3:286–9.
32. Panchbhavi VK, Andersen CR, Vallurupalli S, et al. A minimally disruptive model and three-dimensional evaluation of Lisfranc joint diastasis. J Bone Joint Surg Am 2008;90:2707–13.
33. Lu J, Ebraheim NA, Skie M, et al. Radiographic and computed tomographic evaluation of Lisfranc dislocation: a cadaver study. Foot Ankle Int 1997;18:351–5.
34. Haapamaki V, Kiuru M, Koskinen S. Lisfranc fracture-dislocation in patients with multiple trauma: diagnosis with multidetector computed tomography. Foot Ankle Int 2004;25:614–9.

35. Kalia V, Fishman EK, Carrino JA, et al. Epidemiology, imaging, and treatment of Lisfranc fracture-dislocations revisited. Skeletal Radiol 2012;41:129–36.
36. Richter M, Wippermann B, Krettek C, et al. Fractures and fracture dislocations of the midfoot: occurrence, causes and long-term results. Foot Ankle Int 2001;22:392–8.
37. Hawkes NC, Flemming DJ, Ho VB. Radiology corner. Answer to last month's radiology case and image: subtle Lisfranc injury: low energy midfoot sprain. Mil Med 2007;172:xii–xiii.
38. Hatem SF, Davis A, Sundaram M. Your diagnosis? Midfoot sprain: Lisfranc ligament disruption. Orthopedics 2005;28(2):75–7.
39. Potter HG, Deland JT, Gusmer PB, et al. Magnetic resonance imaging of the Lisfranc ligament of the foot. Foot Ankle Int 1998;19:438–46.
40. Preidler KW, Wang YC, Brossmann J, et al. Tarsometatarsal joint: anatomic details on MR images. Radiology 1996;199:733–6.
41. Raikin SM, Elias I, Dheer S, et al. Prediction of midfoot instability in the subtle Lisfranc injury. Comparison of magnetic resonance imaging with intraoperative findings. J Bone Joint Surg Am 2009;91:892–9.
42. Thompson MC, Mormino MA. Injury to the tarsometatarsal joint complex. J Am Acad Orthop Surg 2003;11:260–7.
43. Calder JD, Whitehouse SL, Saxby TS. Results of isolated Lisfranc injuries and the effect of compensation claims. J Bone Joint Surg Br 2004;86:527–30.
44. Curtis MJ, Myerson M, Szura B. Tarsometatarsal joint injuries in the athlete. Am J Sports Med 1993;21:497–502.
45. Davies MS, Saxby TS. Intercuneiform instability and the "gap" sign. Foot Ankle Int 1999;20:606–9.
46. Kuo RS, Tejwani NC, Digiovanni CW, et al. Outcome after open reduction and internal fixation of Lisfranc joint injuries. J Bone Joint Surg Am 2000;82:1609–18.
47. Ly TV, Coetzee JC. Treatment of primarily ligamentous Lisfranc joint injuries: primary arthrodesis compared with open reduction and internal fixation. A prospective, randomized study. J Bone Joint Surg Am 2006;88:514–20.
48. Rajapakse B, Edwards A, Hong T. A single surgeon's experience of treatment of Lisfranc joint injuries. Injury 2006;37:914–21.
49. Deol R, Roche A, Calder JD. Return to training and playing following acute Lisfranc injury in elite professional soccer and rugby players. Baltimore (MD): American Orthopaedic Society for Sports Medicine; 2012.
50. Arntz CT, Veith RG, Hansen ST Jr. Fractures and fracture-dislocations of the tarsometatarsal joint. J Bone Joint Surg Am 1988;70:173–81.
51. van Rijn J, Dorleijn DM, Boetes B, et al. Missing the Lisfranc fracture: a case report and review of the literature. J Foot Ankle Surg 2012;51:270–4.
52. Perez Blanco R, Rodriguez Merchan C, Canosa Sevillano R, et al. Tarsometatarsal fractures and dislocations. J Orthop Trauma 1988;2:188–94.
53. Tan YH, Chin TW, Mitra AK, et al. Tarsometatarsal (Lisfranc's) injuries—results of open reduction and internal fixation. Ann Acad Med Singapore 1995;24:816–9.
54. Lee CA, Birkedal JP, Dickerson EA, et al. Stabilization of Lisfranc joint injuries: a biomechanical study. Foot Ankle Int 2004;25:365–70.
55. Alberta FG, Aronow MS, Barrero M, et al. Ligamentous Lisfranc joint injuries: a biomechanical comparison of dorsal plate and transarticular screw fixation. Foot Ankle Int 2005;26:462–73.
56. Sangeorzan BJ, Hansen ST Jr. Early and late posttraumatic foot reconstruction. Clin Orthop Relat Res 1989;86–91.

57. Marks RM, Parks BG, Schon LC. Midfoot fusion technique for neuroarthropathic feet: biomechanical analysis and rationale. Foot Ankle Int 1998;19:507–10.
58. Cantu RV, Koval KJ. The use of locking plates in fracture care. J Am Acad Orthop Surg 2006;14:183–90.
59. Thordarson DB, Hedman TP, Gross D, et al. Biomechanical evaluation of polylactide absorbable screws used for syndesmosis injury repair. Foot Ankle Int 1997; 18:622–7.
60. Thordarson DB, Hurvitz G. PLA screw fixation of Lisfranc injuries. Foot Ankle Int 2002;23:1003–7.
61. Brin YS, Nyska M, Kish B. Lisfranc injury repair with the TightRope device: a short-term case series. Foot Ankle Int 2010;31:624–7.
62. Ahmed S, Bolt B, McBryde A. Comparison of standard screw fixation versus suture button fixation in Lisfranc ligament injuries. Foot Ankle Int 2010;31:892–6.
63. Vertullo CJ, Easley ME, Nunley JA. The transverse dorsal approach to the Lisfranc joint. Foot Ankle Int 2002;23:420–6.
64. Mann RA, Prieskorn D, Sobel M. Mid-tarsal and tarsometatarsal arthrodesis for primary degenerative osteoarthrosis or osteoarthrosis after trauma. J Bone Joint Surg Am 1996;78:1376–85.
65. Lui TH. Arthroscopic tarsometatarsal (Lisfranc) arthrodesis. Knee Surg Sports Traumatol Arthrosc 2007;15:671–5.
66. Coetzee JC. Making sense of Lisfranc injuries. Foot Ankle Clin 2008;13:695–704, ix.
67. Mulier T, Reynders P, Dereymaeker G, et al. Severe Lisfranc injuries: primary arthrodesis or ORIF? Foot Ankle Int 2002;23:902–5.
68. Vertullo CJ, Nunley JA. Participation in sports after arthrodesis of the foot or ankle. Foot Ankle Int 2002;23:625–8.
69. Horton GA, Olney BW. Deformity correction and arthrodesis of the midfoot with a medial plate. Foot Ankle 1993;14:493–9.
70. Komenda GA, Myerson MS, Biddinger KR. Results of arthrodesis of the tarsometatarsal joints after traumatic injury. J Bone Joint Surg Am 1996;78:1665–76.
71. Sangeorzan BJ, Veith RG, Hansen ST Jr. Salvage of Lisfranc's tarsometatarsal joint by arthrodesis. Foot Ankle 1990;10:193–200.
72. Johnson JE, Johnson KA. Dowel arthrodesis for degenerative arthritis of the tarsometatarsal (Lisfranc) joints. Foot Ankle 1986;6:243–53.
73. Buzzard BM, Briggs PJ. Surgical management of acute tarsometatarsal fracture dislocation in the adult. Clin Orthop Relat Res 1998;125–33.
74. Sands AK, Grose A. Lisfranc injuries. Injury 2004;35(Suppl 2):SB71–6.

Fifth Metatarsal Fractures in the Athlete: Evidence for Management

Gowreeson Thevendran, MFSEM (UK), FRCS (Tr & Orth)[a,*],
Rupinderbir Singh Deol, MSc, DIC, FRCS (Tr & Orth)[b],
James D.F. Calder, TD, MD, FRCS (Tr & Orth), FFSEM (UK)[c,d]

KEYWORDS

- Fifth metatarsal • Jones fractures • Stress fracture • Athletes

KEY POINTS

- Tuberosity avulsion (zone 1) fractures are successfully treated conservatively.
- Proximal metaphyseal/diaphyseal junction (zone 2) and proximal diaphyseal (zone 3) fractures should be surgically fixed to enable more rapid union and return to sports. Intramedullary screw fixation is supported by level III and IV studies, although no implant has shown superiority and there is insufficient evidence to recommend bone grafting acutely.
- Extracorporeal shock-wave therapy may have a role in treating delayed unions and nonunions, with some encouraging early results, although the evidence is limited.
- Chronic injuries (delayed unions and nonunions) are surgically treated successfully by several techniques, including intramedullary screw fixation, curettage, and bone grafting.

INTRODUCTION

Fifth metatarsal fractures are among the most common forefoot injuries, particularly in the young athletic population, including elite athletes.[1,2] The estimated incidence of these fractures has been recorded as 1.8 per 1000 person-years.[3,4] However, most of the controversy surrounding the treatment of fifth metatarsal fractures relates to those injuries sustained at the proximal aspect. This conundrum is partly perpetuated by a lax application of anatomic terms and usage of eponyms such as Jones fracture.[5,6] Historically, controversy surrounding treatment of fractures in this anatomic location centered around whether treatment should be operative or nonoperative, the role of bone grafting, fixation with an intramedullary screw or other internal fixation devices, and differences in the management of acute and chronic injuries. More recently, there has been an

All authors declare no conflicts of interest in the authorship and publication of this contribution.
[a] Department of Orthopaedics, Tan Tock Seng Hospital, 11 Jalan Tan Tock Seng, Singapore 308433; [b] Lister/QEII Hospitals, East & North Herts NHS Trust, Coreys Mill Lane, Stevenage, Hertfordshire SG1 4AB, UK; [c] Chelsea & Westminster Hospital, 369 Fulham Road, London SW10 9NH, UK; [d] The Fortius Clinic, 17 Fitzhardinge Street, London W1H 6EQ, UK
* Corresponding author.
E-mail address: xanthus23@hotmail.com

Foot Ankle Clin N Am 18 (2013) 237–254
http://dx.doi.org/10.1016/j.fcl.2013.02.005
1083-7515/13/$ – see front matter © 2013 Elsevier Inc. All rights reserved.

foot.theclinics.com

evolving debate on rates and reasons for refracture and whether athletes should be treated any differently than the more sedentary individual sustaining a similar fracture.

Given that much of the interest in the fifth metatarsal surrounds its proximal aspect, this review focuses on the evidence for management of proximal fifth metatarsal fractures. After a brief consideration of the anatomy and biomechanics, the evidence for treatment in the different zones of the proximal fifth metatarsal, the role of recent adjunctive therapies, and differences in the approach to acute and chronic injuries are discussed.

ANATOMY AND BIOMECHANICS

The anatomy and biomechanics of the fifth metatarsal may predispose an athlete involved in running and cutting sports to injure this bone. Inherently strong ligamentous and capsular attachments are present between the fourth and fifth metatarsals and between the fifth metatarsal and the cuboid. These attachments terminate at the metaphyseal-diaphyseal junction. It is these strong attachments that allow stresses at the mobile metatarsal head to be directed to the base of the fifth metatarsal, with the metaphyseal-diaphyseal junction acting as a fulcrum.

Force-plate analysis has shown that a vertical or a medial lateral force typically occurs at the time of fracture.[5] Tuberosity avulsion fractures are typically caused by inversion injuries, although this mechanism does not seem to be a component of injuries that occur distal to the tuberosity.[5] Cadaveric studies suggest that it is the firm attachment of the lateral band of the plantar aponeurosis at the tip of the tuberosity that is responsible for these fractures, rather than the more distal peroneus brevis attachement.[7,8] Gross and Bunch[9] analyzed stresses during running and showed that the highest stresses occurred in the first and second metatarsals. The highest peak force, apart from those at the first and second metatarsals, occurred at the fifth metatarsal. These investigators also noted that the cortical thickness of the fifth metatarsal was the least amongst the 5 metatarsals.

BLOOD SUPPLY

Several publications have reported the relevance of blood supply to the fifth metatarsal with regards to fracture healing.[10,11] In 1927, Carp[12] reported on 21 fractures of the proximal fifth metatarsal and suggested vascular insufficiency as a potential cause for a high incidence of delayed unions in the series. Subsequently, Smith and colleagues[10] described the intraosseous blood supply of the fifth metatarsal from cadaveric dissections. Blood supply originates from 3 potential sources: the nutrient artery, the metaphyseal perforators, and the periosteal arteries. The nutrient artery enters the bone from the medial aspect at the junction of the proximal and middle third of the diaphysis and terminates in linear branches both proximally and distally. The metaphyseal arteries originate from the surrounding soft tissues and penetrate the metaphysis in a random distribution. Therefore, injuries to the proximal diaphysis of the metatarsal are likely to injure the proximal branch of the intraosseous nutrient vessel, thereby impairing the blood supply to the distal portion of the proximal fragment of the bone.

MANAGEMENT OF FIFTH METATARSAL FRACTURES
Introduction

The evolution of the treatment approach to fifth metatarsal fractures in the athlete has been largely influenced by the drive to reduce the time away from sport and ensure reliability of healing. More recently, increasing reports of unacceptably high nonunion rates, refracture rates, and delayed return to activities with nonoperative treatment have provided an impetus for primary fixation as the accepted standard of care for the elite athlete.[5,13,14]

Treatment algorithms for fractures of the fifth metatarsal are largely related to the anatomic location of the fracture. Treatment of lesser metatarsal shaft fractures emphasizes the resting position of the metatarsal heads.[15] Although there is no definitive study describing the millimeter or angular displacement that is acceptable, the criteria most commonly mentioned include less than 10° of angulation or 3 to 4 mm of translation in any plane.[16,17] Moderate displacement in the coronal plane is often well tolerated. However, displacement of any fracture in the sagittal plane alters the weight-bearing characteristics across the metatarsal heads.[18]

In general, an isolated fracture with minimal or no displacement is treated with a hard-sole shoe, an off-the-shelf walker boot, or a short-leg cast, with progressive weight bearing. Patients are then advised to gradually progress to comfortable and well-padded shoes after approximately 4 weeks. Although displacement outside the deformity criteria outlined earlier may warrant closed or open reduction, most diaphyseal and distal fifth metatarsal fractures are amenable to closed reduction and cast immobilization. The failure to achieve closed reduction is an indication for open reduction and internal stabilization with Kirschner wires.[19]

The proximal fifth metatarsal

In 1902, Sir Robert Jones published his original case series "Fracture of the base of the fifth metatarsal bone by indirect violence" in *The Annals of Surgery*.[19] His interest was prompted by a foot injury that he sustained while dancing. His rationale for metatarsal fractures contradicted the consensus of opinion at the time that all metatarsal fractures were caused by direct violence. He reported 6 cases of metatarsal fractures that occurred without direct violence, together with reproductions of the radiographs for each. Although the course of the fracture lines is not distinct given the poor quality of the images, Jones commented that there was little doubt that the fracture was complete.

The first case in Jones' series was his own metatarsal fracture. The published radiograph confirmed a fracture line extending through the lateral cortex in the direction of the proximal portion of the articulation between the fourth and fifth metatarsals. He noted that, when the heel was off the ground, body weight expends itself on the fifth metatarsal, rotating it slightly inward.[19] The strong and complex ligamentous attachments between the fourth and fifth metatarsals made it easier to break the bone rather than dislocate it.[19] It seems that an adductor moment across the relatively fixed fourth and fifth metatarsal base causes an acute fracture of the base of the fifth metatarsal at the area between the insertion of the peroneus brevis and tertius tendons (zone 2).

Another case in Jones' series included a more distal fracture line. Radiographs showed thickening of the cortices and evidence of sclerotic changes within the intramedullary canal. Since the publication of Jones' series, it has been acknowledged that fractures in this region of the metatarsal (zone 3) are often, but not always, stress fractures. Studies have suggested that stress from the lateral aspect of the fifth metatarsal head occurs in zone 3, where repeated varus forces on the distal end of the bone are believed to be responsible for stress fractures.[5,20] Radiographically, these fractures usually open up laterally rather than plantarwards, suggesting that the insulting force vector is more lateral than plantar.[5]

Fracture zones of the proximal fifth metatarsal

Jones's observation at the turn of the century that fractures of the base of the fifth metatarsal can occur as a result of indirect trauma earned him the eponym Jones fracture for fractures at the metaphyseal-diaphyseal junction. However, it was not until 1960, from a series of 46 proximal fifth metatarsal fractures, that Stewart[21] was able to show a difference in mechanism of injury and in the prognosis for "fractures at the juncture of the shaft and base (Jones fracture) and fractures of the styloid process." Ever since, appreciation of different anatomic locations linked to individual mechanisms of injury has paved the way to recognition of prognostic fracture zones of the proximal fifth metatarsal.[22] Recognition of this anatomic classification system has enabled individualized treatment strategies, more meaningful prognoses, and less confusion in the published literature.

The next section discusses the evidence for current treatment strategies in these 3 distinct fracture zones of the proximal fifth metatarsal.

Zone 1 Injuries

Fractures in zone 1 are tuberosity avulsion fractures that usually begin laterally on the tuberosity and extend proximally into the metatarsocuboid joint. These fracture lines typically traverse a segment of cancellous bone that has a good blood supply. These are the most common fractures of the proximal fifth metatarsal.[6]

There are other radiographic appearances that may mimic a tuberosity avulsion fracture. The first instance is a tuberosity apophysis, which may be seen in an adolescent who has sustained an inversion injury to the foot. Another differential diagnosis may be an os perineum, which is typically seen adjacent to the lateral border of the cuboid, within the peroneus longus tendon.

Evidence for treatment

Most of the published literature has cited good success with healing of these fractures.[23,24] The recommended treatment is symptomatic care, with weight bearing as tolerated.[5,6] The patient may be offered a stiff-soled shoe and advised to ice, elevate, and apply a compressive bandage to aid swelling control. Although a functional brace or a short-leg walking cast may be theoretically more comfortable, there is no evidence in the literature to associate the use of such orthoses with decreasing time to union. The literature suggests that most of these fractures heal by either bony union or asymptomatic fibrous union within 6 to 8 weeks.[25,26] Radiographic evidence of union lags significantly behind pain resolution, which remains the more important consideration in these fractures, even in the athletic population.

Historical data have suggested that operative intervention may be indicated in the event of a significant articular step-off (2–3 mm) or large avulsed fragments involving the articular surface with or without a rotatory component.[23,25] In these scenarios, various investigators[26–29] have proposed operative stabilization techniques, including open reduction and internal fixation with an interfragmentary screw or plates, closed reduction, and Kirschner wire fixation or tension band wiring. However, given the scarcity of surgical intervention in these fracture subtypes both in the general and athletic population and the lack of comparative clinical trials, these recommendations are poorly substantiated by evidence in the published literature.

Zone 2 Injuries

Zone 2 corresponds to the metaphyseal-diaphyseal junction, anatomic site of the true Jones fracture. Stewart[21] defined a true Jones fracture as a transverse fracture at the junction of the diaphysis and the metaphysis without extension distal to the fourth to fifth intermetatarsal articulation. The fracture line in zone 2 typically begins laterally in the distal portion of the tuberosity and extends transversely or obliquely into the region of the medial cortex, where the fifth metatarsal articulates with the fourth metatarsal.[25,27]

Athletes who sustain these injuries often describe a large adduction force applied to the forefoot while the ankle is plantar flexed (eg, a pivoting or cutting maneuver in soccer, with most of the body weight on the metatarsal heads).[27] The high load on the plantar aspect of the fifth metatarsal head generates a large bending motion across the relatively fixed fourth and fifth metatarsal bases. This segment of the fifth metatarsal (zone 2) remains relatively immobile in the coronal plane and acts as a fulcrum during adduction of the forefoot, and thus may fracture with large bending moments.

Since first identified, these fractures have been recognized to be associated with delayed union, nonunion, and refracture after healing.[1] This situation poses a difficult problem, particularly to the competitive athlete, for whom an early return to sporting activities is a priority. Furthermore, several studies have suggested that a nonoperative approach with non–weight bearing immobilization may not produce optimal long-term outcomes in this patient cohort.[30–32] This situation has prompted the introduction of various surgical treatment options, in particular the minifragment intramedullary screw fixation. The poor biological potential of this fracture because of its compromised blood supply has also recently been the subject of studies evaluating the role of autogenous bone graft and bone marrow substitutes.

Evidence for choice of management: operative versus nonoperative treatment

Through the 1980s and 1990s, several investigators have debated the role of nonoperative versus operative management in zone 2 fractures. The most noteworthy of these are the studies by Mologne and colleagues[33] and Low and colleagues.[34] In a level I study comparing early screw fixation with casting for acute Jones fractures, Mologne and colleagues compared 2 groups of athletes (n = 37 in total). The patients in the conservative group were immobilized in a cast for 8 weeks and those in the operative group were kept in a splint for a fortnight after screw fixation. The median time to return to sports was 15 weeks in the cast group and 8 weeks in the screw group. These investigators showed a statistically different union rate between the operative group (94%) and the nonoperative group (67%). In a level III study of 86 NFL (National Football League) athletes, Low and colleagues showed a union rate of 94% in their operative series versus 80% in their nonoperative group.

In a recent systematic review (2012) of 21 selected articles discussing treatment of proximal metatarsal fractures in both the athletic and nonathletic population, Kerkhoffs and colleagues[35] concluded that nonoperative treatment of Jones fractures resulted in a longer time to union and a higher number of delayed unions or nonunions compared with operative treatment. Given the higher healing rate, faster time to union, and a faster return to sports, most investigators now advocate surgical treatment of acute zone 2 fractures in the athlete.

Evidence for the type of surgical fixation

The pursuit of rapid and predictable results has led to surgical intervention, with intramedullary screw fixation being the popular surgical technique of choice in the athletic population. Advocates for this technique have suggested individualized screw dimensions to achieve greatest possible mechanical compression across the fracture site, emphasizing the need to conserve the local biology through a percutaneous entry point.

There is an evolving body of level III and level IV evidence in favor of intramedullary screw fixation for zone 2 fractures in the athletic patient (**Fig. 1**).[13,33,36] Porter and colleagues[30] reported on 23 consecutive acute Jones fractures in athletes treated with 4.5-mm cannulated screws and 1 week in crutches. The radiological union was

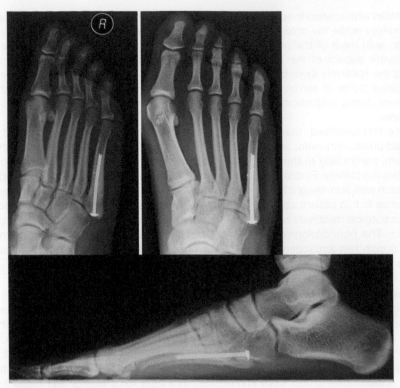

Fig. 1. Anteroposterior/oblique/lateral radiographs showing union 3 months after intramedullary screw fixation for an acute zone 2 fracture. Note the bend of titanium 4-mm cannulated screw in the narrow medullary canal.

99% and the mean time return to sports was 7.5 weeks. Chuckpaiwong and colleagues[36] retrospectively reported on a series of 32 zone 2 (27 athletes) and 29 zone 3 (25 athletes) fractures. Competitive athletes treated with an intramedullary screw reported a significantly quicker time to return to sports (15.3 vs 30.0 weeks) compared with those treated nonoperatively.

Nevertheless, there have been a few reported series of failures with intramedullary screw fixation of proximal fifth metatarsal fractures in terms of refracture or screw breakage. Wright and colleagues[37] reported on 6 refractures after cannulated screw fixation of Jones fractures in athletes (screw sizes ranging from 4 mm to 5 mm). Despite both clinical and radiographic union, 3 patients sustained a refracture the day after return to full activity, and 3 other patients experienced a refracture within 4.5 months after return to activity. Larson and colleagues,[38] in their series of 15 cannulated screw fixations of Jones fractures, reported 4 refractures and 2 symptomatic nonunions. Both groups of investigators concluded that premature return to full activity may increase the risk of procedural failure. Furthermore, a larger-diameter screw should be considered for patients with a larger body mass, and functional bracing or modified footwear should be recommended to facilitate return to play.

Although the cannulated 4.5-mm partially threaded cancellous stainless steel screw seems to be the common surgical choice, there has been some controversy on the choice of screw diameter, length, and material. However, there is insufficient evidence to suggest that 1 screw type is superior to another.

Evidence for bone grafting with operative fixation
The argument for bone grafting fractures of the fifth metatarsal base first arose after Dameron's[39] series in 1975 of 20 proximal fifth metatarsal diaphyseal fractures. The investigator showed 5 cases of nonunion that were treated with sliding bone grafts and advocated bone grafting of all proximal diaphyseal fractures, especially in athletes. Ever since, many investigators have advocated the use of bone grafts, mainly in the setting of zone 3 injuries and chronic proximal fifth metatarsal fractures.[13,32,40]

However, more recently, given the morbidity associated with iliac crest bone graft harvest, clinical studies have focused on the efficacy of autologous bone marrow aspirate (BMA) for the treatment of difficult fractures.[41,42] However, there has been little published evidence on the isolated role of bone grafting in proximal fifth metatarsal fractures. Hunt and Anderson[43] retrospectively reviewed 21 elite athletes who had undergone revision fixation of a Jones fracture nonunion with intramedullary screw fixation and autologous bone grafting. Twenty patients in the series had either (1) iliac crest cancellous bone graft or (2) BMA + demineralized bone matrix (DBM). These investigators concluded that there was no significant difference in time to radiographic healing or return to sport when comparing cancellous bone graft with BMA+DBM. Murawski and Kennedy[44] reported on the results of 26 consecutive athletes with acute proximal fifth metatarsal fractures (17 zone 2 and 9 zone 3 fractures) undergoing percutaneous internal fixation with an individualized-diameter partially threaded non-cannulated screw and autologous BMA. These investigators reported a 96% radiological union rate as evaluated by standard radiographs at 8 weeks after intervention and a mean time returning to sporting activities of 7.6 weeks.

There is insufficient evidence to recommend bone grafting in the setting of acute zone 2 injuries. Further randomized controlled trials are needed before their role as a therapeutic adjunct in the athletic population can be established.

Zone 3 Injuries

Injuries in the proximal diaphyseal region are typically stress fractures, as mentioned earlier, although they may be confused with delayed unions and nonunions. They are common injuries in the athlete. Ekstrand and Torstveit[45] prospectively followed 2379 elite male footballers over 8 years, finding 51 stress fractures, the fifth metatarsal being the commonest (78%). Younger age and intensive preseason training were implicated as risk factors. Biomechanical work has also shown that the greatest pressure differential between the base and head occurs during acceleration, so adequate rest between bouts of acceleration during training may have preventative value.[46] Clinical assessment should include a careful search for underlying risk factors, including nutritional and hormonal issues, and should explore training techniques and methods.[47,48] Athletic stress fractures may be missed on initial examination,[49] and a high index of suspicion should be maintained[50] and further imaging (computed tomography [CT] or magnetic resonance imaging) obtained if necessary to enable early detection.[47,51]

In 1984, Torg and colleagues[32] reported a series of 46 proximal fifth metatarsal fractures and guidelines for nonsurgical and surgical management. Fractures of the proximal part of the diaphysis were classified into 3 types: acute fracture lacking sclerosis (I), delayed union with fracture line widening and presence of intramedullary sclerosis (II), and nonunion with complete obliteration of the medullary canal with sclerotic bone (III).

Evidence for choice of management: operative versus nonoperative treatment
Zogby and Baker[52] retrospectively evaluated nonoperative treatment in 10 patients using a short-legged non–weight bearing cast, until radiographic and clinical union followed by 6 weeks of limited activity. However, the group was heterogeneous, with

3 acute injuries in nonathletes and the remainder were chronic injuries in athletes. Mean time to radiographic and clinical union was 9.4 weeks in the athletic group, and all returned to their preinjury competition level by an average of 12 weeks, whereas the acute fractures in the nonathletes took more than double the time to heal.

Length of healing time, nonunion, and concerns of refracture have been the impetus for fixation. Nonoperative treatment has been associated with a higher rate of treatment failure,[53,54] and early fixation in the athlete is widely supported.[13,39,50,53–55]

Evidence for the type of surgical fixation

DeLee and colleagues[13] reported a series of 10 athletes treated with closed intramedullary screw fixation, with union at an average of 7.5 weeks and return to sport in an average of 8.5 weeks. Although 7 of 10 required shoe modifications for pain over the screw head, there were no refractures. Pecina and colleagues[54] have reported long-term follow-up of 20 top-level athletes treated with intramedullary screw fixation, using American Orthopaedic Foot and Ankle Society midfoot score and pedobarographic analysis. Clinical union was achieved in 95%, with only 1 refracture. Twelve athletes attained higher levels of training, although 1 failed to make the preinjury level.

In Pecina and colleagues' series,[54] 18 of the group presented with varus of the metatarsus and the midfoot and were recommended orthotic use during their competitive careers. However, Hestsroni and colleagues[56] examined 10 professional soccer players who returned to professional activity after a unilateral fifth metatarsal stress fracture. These investigators aimed to assess whether those who sustained this injury had an exceptional static foot structure or dynamic loading pattern. Injured, contralateral, and control feet were assessed. The findings showed no exceptional static foot structure, and dynamically, there was lateral metatarsal unloading, which may be pathogenic or adaptive. The investigators concluded that orthotic use ought to be tailored, focusing on individual dynamic evaluation rather than static foot and arch characteristics.

Lee and colleagues[57] retrospectively reviewed 42 patients with acute (Torg I) and chronic (Torg II) fractures treated with modified tension band wiring using 2 cortical screws. CT evaluation revealed a mean time to union of 75 days (40–150 days), with all patients returning to previous sporting activity, although there were 4 refractures, 4 delayed unions, and 1 nonunion.

Evidence for bone grafting with operative fixation

Autologous cancellous bone grafting combined with intramedullary screw fixation has been proposed. Popovic and colleagues[58] treated 18 high-level soccer players, 11 with a percutaneous screw and 7 with an open approach using autologous cancellous bone grafting along with screw fixation. Although all cases united and returned to full sports by 12 weeks, 3 players in the percutaneously fixed group refractured at 4.5, 5.2, and 6.0 months after surgery. These fractures were all revised with open curettage, autologous grafting, and rescrew fixation and none subsequently refractured.

BMAs may have a role, although they do require further evaluation. Murawski and Kennedy[44] reported on 26 athletes, 9 of whom were zone 3 injuries, using a fracture-specific percutaneous screw system and BMA, with a mean overall time to union of 5 weeks (range 5–24 weeks).

There is insufficient evidence to advocate primary bone grafting of acute zone 3 fractures.

Shock-Wave Therapy and Electromagnetic Fields

Shock-wave therapy

Extracorporeal shock-wave therapy (ECSWT) is increasingly used in the in the treatment of foot and ankle tendinopathies and fasciopathies. Evidence is emerging that it may have a role in treating bony disease, namely stress fractures,[59] delayed unions, and nonunions,[60,61] and possibly acute fractures,[62] although further research is required to provide accurate union rates.[63] Much of the literature relates to long bone nonunions.[64] Although the mechanism of action in musculoskeletal disorders remains largely unknown, based on animal models, it is believed that the high-energy acoustic waves induce neovascularization, which increases cell proliferation and eventually tissue regeneration.[65] Its use offers numerous advantages to surgery, being noninvasive, well tolerated, and yielding few complications.[66]

Furia and colleagues[67] reviewed its use in zone 2 nonunions, comparing 2 groups (23 cases treated with high-energy shock wave and 23 cases with intramedullary screw fixation). At 3 months after intervention, union occurred in 20 cases in the shock-wave group and 18 in the screw fixation group. At 6 months, 1 further case of union had occurred in the shock-wave group. Whereas the shock-wave group had 1 complication with petechiae, there were 11 complications in the screw fixation group (1 refracture, 1 cellulitis, and 9 cases of symptomatic hardware).

Alvarez and colleagues[68] evaluated shock-wave treatment of nonunion and delayed union in 34 proximal metatarsal fractures with a single-arm multicenter study. Although the group was heterogeneous, containing fractures of metatarsals 1 to 4 and zone 2 fifth metatarsal fractures, most (25) were in the latter group. Application was performed under general or regional anesthesia. These investigators showed a success rate of 71% at 12 weeks after treatment. The commonest side effect attributable to the treatment was swelling. The patients were not all athletes and the age range was 16 to 75 years.

Studies of athletes include one by Moretti and colleagues,[59] who reported their experience of 10 soccer players treated with chronic fifth metatarsal or tibial stress fracture treated with 3 to 4 sessions of low-energy to middle-energy ECSWT, which enabled all players to gradually return to sport. At mean follow-up of 8 weeks, there was 100% union. Taki and colleagues[69] treated 5 stress fractures in athletes, 1 of which was a fifth metatarsal, with a single high-energy focused treatment. All achieved radiographic union in 2 to 3.5 months and returned to sport 3.5 to 6 months after treatment. Albisetti and colleagues[70] treated stress fractures of the second and third metatarsals in 18 young trainee ballet dancers with shock- wave therapy and 1 with pulsed electromagnetic fields combined with rest. All had good results, with short times to return to dancing without pain. Luthe and Nurmi-Lüthje[71] reported a single case of a high-level soccer player with a proximal fifth metatarsal delayed union treated with low-intensity pulsed ultrasonographic treatment for 3 months. The investigators suggested that this treatment may accelerate time return to sport.

Although there may be a place for shock-wave therapy in the management of proximal fifth metatarsal fractures in the athlete, this lacks strong evidence and requires more research.[72]

Electromagnetic bone stimulation

Although some level IV studies support the use of electrical bone stimulation in the arthrodesis nonunion setting, there is little to justify its use in the treatment of fresh fractures.[73] Holmes[74] treated 9 delayed unions and nonunion of the fifth metatarsal with pulsed electromagnetic fields and a non–weight bearing cast, with union in a mean time of 4 months (2–8 months). Benazzo and colleagues[75] treated 25 lower limb stress fractures, including fifth metatarsal fractures, in athletes with application of a sinusoidal wave alternate current, with a mean stimulation time of 52 days. Twenty-two fractures united. There may be a role for electromagnetic bone stimulation as an adjunct to surgery in the athlete, although evidence is still lacking.

Chronic Fractures

Delayed and nonunion of the fifth metatarsal fractures may compromise time to return to sport and thereby have a profound impact on an athlete's career. Hence, surgical intervention is usually necessary in both zone 2[23] and 3[76] nonunions in the athlete. The evidence for management largely comprises level IV studies. Several of the studies include groups of both delayed and nonunions together, but often differentiate between them.[30,32,74,77,78]

Delayed unions

Although cases of delayed union treated conservatively may eventually unite, this may require long periods, so early surgery is generally recommended in athletes.[32,79] Intramedullary screw fixation seems to be a common method of fixation, with or without grafting.

Nonoperative management Torg and colleagues[32] evaluated 46 fractures distal to the tuberosity, of which 12 were delayed union characterized by a previous injury or fracture, fracture line involving both cortices with associated new periosteal bone formation, a widened fracture line with adjacent radiolucency caused by bone resorption, and evidence of intramedullary sclerosis. Of the 12, 10 were initially treated with plaster cast immobilization and weight bearing, of which 7 healed at a mean of 15.1 months and 3 required grafting for nonunion. These 3 nonunions and another delayed union that was treated surgically with grafting primarily all healed within 12 weeks. These investigators advocated that active athletes benefit from medullary curettage and bone grafting, although delayed unions may be treated conservatively.[32]

Khan and colleagues[78] retrospectively evaluated fractures distal to the tuberosity, of which 15 were nonunions treated nonoperatively. These investigators showed that although these fractures may eventually unite, this may take up to 20 weeks, thereby supporting the role for early surgery in athletes. Holmes[74] treated 5 delayed unions in his group, along with 4 nonunions using pulsed electromagnetic fields. The union rate was slow in this subgroup, with a mean of 14.4 weeks.

Intramedullary screw fixation Porter and colleagues[30] used a 4.5-mm cannulated screw without bone grafting to fix 23 consecutive athletes with zone 2 injuries. Casts were not used postoperatively but early mobilization within a boot was permitted. Ten of the series were delayed unions as per Torg and colleagues'[32] classification. Clinical union was 100%, and radiological union assessed by an independent radiologist was 100% in 8 of these cases and 98% and 99% in the other 2. Further, mean time to return to sport was 7.5 weeks in the absence of complications.

Larson and colleagues[38] analyzed cannulated screw fixation of proximal diaphyseal fractures in a series of 15 patients, 7 of whom had delayed unions. Although 3 of these patients went on to uncomplicated union in an average of 9 weeks, 3 of the remaining 4 refractured, requiring further treatment, and 1 went on to nonunion. All of those in whom treatment failed were elite athletes. Portland and colleagues[79] evaluated acute intramedullary screw fixation in a series comprising acute zone 2 injuries, acute proximal diaphyseal fractures, and delayed unions (Torg type I and II, respectively). All 7 of the delayed unions went on to union within 7 to 12 weeks (mean 8.3 weeks).

Tension band wiring Sarimo and colleagues[77] evaluated tension band wiring of 27 zone 2 injuries in mostly high-level athletes that had not united, 25 of which had initial conservative cast treatment and 15 of which lacked intramedullary sclerosis and were deemed delayed unions. These investigators found that all their patients returned to full activity in 8 to 20 weeks, with a mean time to radiographic union of 12.8 weeks.

Nonunions

Shock-wave therapy[66] and pulsed electromagnetic fields[80] have been used to treat nonunions, but surgical treatment remains the standard, either with closed intramedullary screw fixation or autogenous corticocancellous bone grafting.[25]

Intramedullary screw fixation

Intramedullary screw fixation is the commonest type of fixation for nonunions, although it is not without complications (**Figs. 2–5**).

Habbu and colleagues[81] reported that closed intramedullary screw fixation resulted in radiological union in all 14 cases in their series, with a mean time to union of 13.3 weeks (range 8–20 weeks) and unassisted full pain-free weight bearing at 10.2 weeks. One deep infection and 1 sural neuroma were reported. Porter and colleagues'[14] series of 24 consecutive athletes contained 11 zone 2 nonunions treated with 4.5-mm cannulated screw fixation. These investigators reported clinical and radiological union in all cases, with a mean time return to sport for the entire group ranging from 10 days to 12 weeks. Porter and colleagues[82] reported a further study in 2009 treating 20 athletes with zone 2 injuries, 4 of which were nonunions, treated with a 5.5-mm screw. Clinical union occurred in all cases and there was

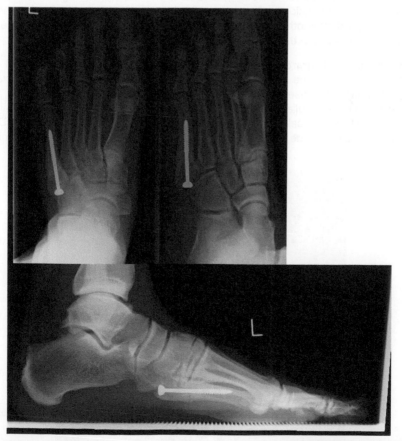

Fig. 2. Anteroposterior/oblique/lateral radiographs of fracture nonunion 1 year after initial fixation with a malleolar screw (patient playing international rugby but with continuing pain at the fracture site).

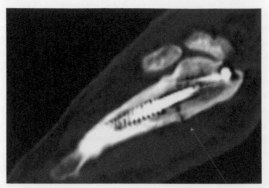

Fig. 3. CT scan confirming fracture nonunion at 1 year after initial screw fixation.

an overall radiographic union of 96.7%. Three refractures occurred, although it is unclear whether these were in the nonunion group.

Furia and colleagues[67] compared the treatment of zone 2 nonunions with intramedullary screw fixation and high-energy shock-wave therapy, finding that both were effective at achieving union by 3 months (18/20 screw, 20/23 shock wave), although this was longer than in other studies. There was also a higher complication rate and slower return to sport in the screw group.

Screw fixation with graft Hunt and Anderson[43] retrospectively evaluated 21 elite athletes treated for zone 2 nonunions or refractures. Intramedullary screw fixation was performed in all cases after curettage at the fracture site, reverse drilling, then tapping of the intramedullary canal. Eight cases were treated with autologous cancellous iliac crest graft, 4 calcaneal bone graft, a further 8 had BMA mixed with DBM, 1 patient had DBM alone, and 1 had no graft. Screw sizes varied from 4.5 mm to

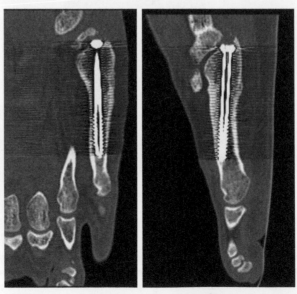

Fig. 4. CT scan confirming bony union at 12 weeks after revision screw fixation with debridement and autologous bone grafting of fracture nonunion.

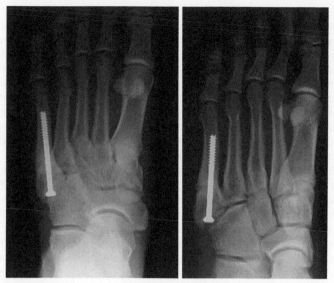

Fig. 5. Anteroposterior/oblique radiographs at 1 year after revision fracture fixation.

6.5 mm solid screws, depending on torque during tapping. All cases united and athletes returned to their preinjury level of activity at a mean of 12.3 weeks (6–16 weeks). One refracture occurred in the series. The investigators advocate use of a large solid screw of 5.5 mm diameter or larger with autologous bone grafting in revision fixation of the nonunion.

Bone grafting Within their series of 46 patients, Torg and colleagues[32] treated 9 nonunions of fractures distal to the tuberosity with resection of bone at the fracture site, medullary curettage, and 2.0-cm by 0.7-cm corticocancellous bone grafts harvested from the distal end of the tibia carefully contoured to prevent occlusion of the fifth metatarsal canal. The resected metatarsal bone was inserted into the tibial harvest site. Eight of the 9 united in a mean of 12.2 weeks (range 10–16 weeks), with 1 continued nonunion occurring in a noncompliant patient who disregarded instructions not to weight bear postoperatively. Hens and Marten[80] also reported union in all 4 cases of nonunion in their series, using an asymmetrical trapezoid autograft.

Tension band wiring Sarimo and colleagues[77] have successfully treated 7 cases with medullary sclerosis and so deemed nonunions in their group of 27 zone 2 injuries with a figure of 8 tension band wiring. All these cases united clinically and radiographically by 15 weeks, with a return to sport between 12 and 20 weeks.

ECSWT and electromagnetic fields In addition to Furia's work with shock-wave therapy, Holmes[74] used pulsed electromagnetic fields and a non–weight bearing cast to successfully treat a group of 9 patients with delayed and nonunions with a mean union time 3 months with no refractures.

MANAGEMENT OF THE ACUTE ZONE 2 FRACTURES AND STRESS FRACTURES IN THE ATHLETE: OUR PREFERRED TECHNIQUE

Percutaneous intramedullary fixation with a 4.5-mm to 5-mm screw is advocated in the acute setting. In those oversized athletes in whom there is a very wide intramedullary canal, a 6.5-mm screw may occasionally be chosen, but the screw head should be buried to ensure that there is no irritation of the peroneus brevis tendon or the cuboid-metatarsal joint. A 1.6-mm Kirchner wire is passed along the intramedullary canal initially under fluoroscopic control to ensure that an optimal entry point is chosen (usually just dorsal to the proximal tip of the tuberosity of the fifth metatarsal. A cannulated drill is then used to ream the entry point, and the Kirschner wire can then be turned round, with the blunt end inserted and tapped down the intramedullary canal to ensure that the point does not perforate the cortex of the shaft; once this has passed the fracture site, the canal is then reamed, the distal canal tapped and the screw inserted, ensuring good compression at the fracture site. If there is poor purchase in the distal metatarsal, a larger-diameter screw is chosen.

In stress fractures in which there is pain and marked cortical thickening, a similar technique is performed. If there is a significant break in the cortex on the plantar-lateral tension side, then the fracture site is routinely opened, the sclerotic bone debrided, and autograft bone graft packed into the fracture site, with the intramedullary screw being used to support the fracture during healing.

Postoperatively, nonsteroidal antiinflammatory drugs are discouraged for 12 weeks and patients are mobilized in a removable boot non–weight bearing for 1 week, partial weight bearing for 2 weeks, and then weight bearing as able in the boot until 6 weeks. There is constant debate as to when it is safe to allow the elite athlete to return to full sports. Most published series suggest 3 months as an appropriate time frame, but undoubtedly refracture is a risk even with radiographic union. Larson and colleagues[38] reported an increased risk of failure of fixation in those returning to sport within 9 weeks, and 83% of the failures were in elite athletes in whom there was pressure to return to sport as soon as possible. Wright and colleagues[37] described 6 refractures in athletes returning at a mean of 8.5 weeks despite previously having clinical and radiographic union. They recommended using a larger screw in larger patients, orthoses postoperatively, and routine use of CT to confirm union in the elite athlete before returning to full sporting activities. We therefore recommend a radiograph at 6 weeks to ensure that there is no separation at the fracture site; the boot may be removed and impact activities are introduced as symptoms allow. A CT scan is routinely performed at 10 weeks, with an expected return to sport at 10 to 12 weeks.

SUMMARY

Fifth metatarsal fractures are common injuries in the athlete, with proximal injuries being the focus of most interest. The main goals of treatment in this population are to ensure rapid union and return to sport at the same or improved level of competition. Descriptive inconsistencies are apparent in the literature. There are 3 anatomic zones of injury in the proximal fifth metatarsal, with differing management strategies: tuberosity avulsion fractures (zone 1), fractures at the metadiaphyseal junction (zone 2), and those in the proximal diaphysis (zone 3). Most zone 1 injuries are successfully treated conservatively, with bony union or symptomatic fibrous union in 6 to 8 weeks. Fixation of displaced fragments may be performed, although it is poorly substantiated by the literature. Surgical fixation yields increased and more rapid union and return to sports in zone 2 injuries. Intramedullary screw fixation is supported by level III and IV studies, although no implant has shown superiority and there is insufficient evidence to recommend bone grafting in this setting. Intramedullary fixation is not without complication. Surgical fixation of zone 3 injuries is well supported by level IV studies, and intramedullary screw fixation has yielded good results. Bone graft application in the acute setting shows no clear superiority. In the chronic injury, good results have been shown with intramedullary screw fixation (both with and without bone grafting), surgical debridement and bone grafting alone, and tension band wiring. Shock-wave therapy and pulsed electromagnetic fields may have a place in the chronic and possibly the acute injury, although the evidence for this is limited.

REFERENCES

1. Raikin SM, Slenker N, Ratigan B. The association of a varus hindfoot and fracture of the fifth metatarsal metaphyseal-diaphyseal junction: the Jones fracture. Am J Sports Med 2008;36(7):1367–72.
2. Vorlat P, Achtergael W, Haentjens P. Predictors of outcome of non-displaced fractures of the base of the fifth metatarsal. Int Orthop 2007;31(1):5–10.
3. Harmath C, Demos TC, Lomasney L, et al. Stress fracture of the fifth metatarsal. Orthopaedics 2001;24:204–8.
4. Hasselman CT, Vogt MT, Stone KL, et al. Foot and ankle fractures in elderly white women. Incidence and risk factors. J Bone Joint Surg Am 2003;85-A:820–4.
5. Kavanaugh JH, Brower TD, Mann RV. The Jones fracture revisited. J Bone Joint Surg Am 1978;60:776–82.
6. Lawrence SJ, Botte MJ. Jones fractures and related fractures of the proximal fifth metatarsal. Foot Ankle Surg 1993;14(6):358–65.
7. Pritsch M, Heim M, Tauber H, et al. An unusual fracture of the base of the fifth metatarsal bone. J Trauma 1980;20(6):530–1.
8. Richli WR, Rosenthal DI. Avulsion fracture of the fifth metatarsal: experimental study of the pathomechanics. Am J Roentgenol 1984;143:889–91.
9. Gross TS, Bunch RP. A mechanical model of metatarsal stress fracture during distance running. Am J Sports Med 1989;17:669–74.
10. Smith JW, Arnoczky SP, Hersh A. The intraosseous blood supply of the fifth metatarsal: implications for proximal fracture healing. Foot Ankle 1992;13:143–52.
11. Shereff MJ, Yang QM, Kummer FJ, et al. Vascular anatomy of the fifth metatarsal. Foot Ankle 1991;11:350–3.
12. Carp L. Fracture of the fifth metatarsal bone with special reference to delayed union. Ann Surg 1927;86:308–20.
13. DeLee JC, Evans JP, Julian J. Stress fracture of the fifth metatarsal. Am J Sports Med 1983;11(5):349–53.
14. Porter DA, Rund AM, Dobslaw R, et al. Comparison of 4.5 and 5.5 mm cannulated stainless steel screw in the competitive and recreational athlete: a clinical and radiographic evaluation. Am J Sports Med 2005;33(5):726–33.
15. Early JS. Fractures and dislocations of the midfoot and forefoot. In: Buckholz RW, Heckman JD, editors. Fractures in adults. 5th edition. Philadelphia: Lippincott Williams & Wilkins; 2001. p. 2215–28.
16. Shereff MJ. Complex fractures of the metatarsals. Orthopaedics 1990;13:875–82.
17. Schenck RC, Heckman JD. Fractures and dislocations of the forefoot: operative and non-operative treatment. J Am Acad Orthop Surg 1995;3(2):70–8.
18. Armagon OE, Shereff MJ. Injuries to the toes and metatarsals. Orthop Clin North Am 2001;32(1):1–10.
19. Jones R. Fracture of the base of the fifth metatarsal bone by indirect violence. Ann Surg 1902;35:697–700.
20. Byrd T. Jones fracture: relearning an old injury. South Med J 1992;85:748–50.
21. Stewart IM. Jones fracture: fracture of the base of fifth metatarsal. Clin Orthop 1960;16:190–8.

22. Den Hartog BD. Fracture of the proximal fifth metatarsal. J Am Acad Orthop Surg 1995;3:110–4.
23. Rettig AC, Shelbourne KD, Wilckens J. The surgical treatment of symptomatic nonunions of the proximal (metaphyseal) fifth metatarsal in athletes. Am J Sports Med 1992;20:50–4.
24. Josefsson PO, Karlsson M, Redlund-Johnell I, et al. Closed treatment of Jones fracture: good results in 40 cases after 11-26 years. Acta Orthop Scand 1994; 65:545–7.
25. Rosenberg GA, Sferra JJ. Treatment strategies for acute fractures and nonunions of the proximal fifth metatarsal. J Am Acad Orthop Surg 2000;8(5):332–8.
26. Dameron TB. Fractures of the proximal fifth metatarsal: selecting the best treatment option. J Am Acad Orthop Surg 1995;3(2):110–4.
27. Quill GE. Fractures of the proximal fifth metatarsal. Orthop Clin North Am 1995; 26(2):353–61.
28. Zwitser EW, Breederveld RS. Fractures of the fifth metatarsal: diagnosis and treatment. Injury 2010;41:555–62.
29. Giordano AR, Fallat LM. Strength analysis of intraosseous wire fixation for avulsion fractures of the fifth metatarsal base. J Foot Ankle Surg 2004;43:225–30.
30. Porter DA, Duncan M, Meyer SJ. Fifth metatarsal Jones fracture fixation with a 4.5mm-cannulated stainless steel screw in the competitive and recreational athlete: a clinical and radiographic evaluation. Am J Sports Med 2005;33(5): 726–33.
31. Clapper MF, O'Brien TJ, Lyons PM. Fractures of the fifth metatarsal: analysis of a fracture registry. Clin Orthop Relat Res 1995;315:238–41.
32. Torg JS, Balduini FC, Zelko RR, et al. Fractures of the base of the fifth metatarsal distal to the tuberosity: classification and guidelines for non-surgical and surgical management. J Bone Joint Surg Am 1984;66:209–14.
33. Mologne TS, Lundeen JM, Clapper MF, et al. Early screw fixation versus casting in the treatment of acute Jones fractures. Am J Sports Med 2005;33:970–5.
34. Low K, Noblin JD, Browne JE, et al. Jones fractures in the elite football player. J Surg Orthop Adv 2004;13:156–60.
35. Kerkhoffs GM, Versteegh VE, Sierevelt IN, et al. Treatment of proximal metatarsal V fractures in athletes and non-athletes. Br J Sports Med 2012;46(9):644–8.
36. Chuckpaiwong B, Queen RM, Easley ME, et al. Distinguishing Jones and proximal diaphyseal fractures of the fifth metatarsal. Clin Orthop Relat Res 2008; 466:1966–70.
37. Wright RW, Fischer DA, Shively RA, et al. Refracture of proximal fifth metatarsal (Jones) fracture after intramedullary screw fixation in athletes. Am J Sports Med 2000;28(5):732–6.
38. Larson CM, Almekinders LC, Taft TN, et al. Intramedullary screw fixation of Jones fractures: analysis of failure. Am J Sports Med 2000;30(1):55–60.
39. Dameron TB. Fractures and anatomical variations of the proximal portion of the fifth metatarsal. J Bone Joint Surg Am 1975;57:788–92.
40. Zelko R, Torg J, Rachun A. Proximal diaphyseal fractures of the fifth metatarsal: treatment of the fractures and their complications in athletes. Am J Sports Med 1979;7:95–101.
41. Connolly JF. Injectable bone marrow preparations to stimulate osteogenic repair. Clin Orthop Relat Res 1995;313:8–18.
42. Hernigou P, Mathieu G, Poignard A, et al. Percutaneous autologous bone-marrow grafting for nonunions: surgical technique. J Bone Joint Surg Am 2006; 88(Suppl 1 Pt 2):322–7.

43. Hunt KJ, Anderson RB. Treatment of Jones fracture nonunions and refractures in the elite athlete: outcomes of intramedullary screw fixation with bone grafting. Am J Sports Med 2011;39(9):1948–54.
44. Murawski CD, Kennedy JG. Percutaneous internal fixation of proximal fifth metatarsal fractures (zones II and III) with Charlotte Carolina screw and bone marrow aspirate concentrate: an outcome study in athletes. Am J Sports Med 2011;39(6): 1295–301.
45. Ekstrand J, Torstveit MK. Stress fractures in elite male football players. Scand J Med Sci Sports 2012;22(3):341–6.
46. Orendurff MS, Rohr ES, Segal AD, et al. Biomechanical analysis of stresses to the fifth metatarsal bone during sports maneuvers: implications for fifth metatarsal fractures. Phys Sportsmed 2009;37(2):87–92.
47. Goulart M, O'Malley MJ, Hodgkins CW, et al. Foot and ankle fractures in dancers. Clin Sports Med 2008;27(2):295–304.
48. Monteleone GP Jr. Stress fractures in the athlete. Orthop Clin North Am 1995; 26(3):423–32.
49. Gehrmann RM, Rajan S, Patel DV, et al. Athletes' ankle injuries: diagnosis and management. Am J Orthop (Belle Mead NJ) 2005;34(11):551–61.
50. Brockwell J, Yeung Y, Griffith JF. Stress fractures of the foot and ankle. Sports Med Arthrosc 2009;17(3):149–59.
51. Niva MH, Sormaala MJ, Kiuru MJ, et al. Bone stress injuries of the ankle and foot: an 86-month magnetic resonance imaging-based study of physically active young adults. Am J Sports Med 2007;35(4):643–9.
52. Zogby RG, Baker BE. A review of nonoperative treatment of Jones' fracture. Am J Sports Med 1987;15(4):304–7.
53. Polzer H, Polzer S, Mutschler W, et al. Acute fractures to the proximal fifth metatarsal bone: development of classification and treatment recommendations based on the current evidence. Injury 2012;43(10):1626–32.
54. Pecina M, Bojanic I, Smoljanovic T, et al. Surgical treatment of diaphyseal stress fractures of the fifth metatarsal in competitive athletes: long-term follow-up and computerized pedobarographic analysis. J Am Podiatr Med Assoc 2011; 101(6):517–22.
55. Weinfeld SB, Haddad SL, Myerson MS. Metatarsal stress fractures [review]. Clin Sports Med 1997;16(2):319–38.
56. Hetsroni I, Nyska M, Ben-Sira D, et al. Analysis of foot structure in athletes sustaining proximal fifth metatarsal stress fracture. Foot Ankle Int 2010;31(3): 203–11.
57. Lee KT, Park YU, Young KW, et al. Surgical results of 5th metatarsal stress fracture using modified tension band wiring. Knee Surg Sports Traumatol Arthrosc 2011;19(5):853–7.
58. Popovic N, Jalali A, Georis P, et al. Proximal fifth metatarsal diaphyseal stress fracture in football players. Foot Ankle Surg 2005;11(3):135–41.
59. Moretti B, Notarnicola A, Garofalo R, et al. Shock waves in the treatment of stress fractures. Ultrasound Med Biol 2009;35(6):1042–9.
60. Birnbaum K, Wirtz DC, Siebert CH, et al. Use of extracorporeal shock-wave therapy (ESWT) in the treatment of non-unions. A review of the literature. Arch Orthop Trauma Surg 2002;122(6):324–30.
61. Zelle BA, Gollwitzer H, Zlowodzki M, et al. Extracorporeal shock wave therapy: current evidence. J Orthop Trauma 2010;24(Suppl 1):S66–70.
62. Moretti B, Notarnicola A, Moretti L, et al. Bone healing induced by ESWT. Clin Cases Miner Bone Metab 2009;6(2):155–8.

63. Petrisor B, Lisson S, Sprague S. Extracorporeal shockwave therapy: a systematic review of its use in fracture management. Indian J Orthop 2009;43(2):161–7.
64. Cacchio A, Giordano L, Colafarina O, et al. Extracorporeal shock-wave therapy compared with surgery for hypertrophic long-bone nonunions [Erratum in: J Bone Joint Surg Am 2010;92(5):1241]. J Bone Joint Surg Am 2009;91(11): 2589–97.
65. Wang CJ. An overview of shock wave therapy in musculoskeletal disorders. Chang Gung Med J 2003;26(4):220–32.
66. Furia JP, Rompe JD, Cacchio A, et al. Shock wave therapy as a treatment of nonunions, avascular necrosis, and delayed healing of stress fractures. Foot Ankle Clin 2010;15(4):651–62.
67. Furia JP, Juliano PJ, Wade AM, et al. Shock wave therapy compared with intramedullary screw fixation for nonunion of proximal fifth metatarsal metaphyseal-diaphyseal fractures. J Bone Joint Surg Am 2010;92(4):846–54.
68. Alvarez RG, Cincere B, Channappa C, et al. Extracorporeal shock wave treatment of non- or delayed union of proximal metatarsal fractures. Foot Ankle Int 2011; 32(8):746–54.
69. Taki M, Iwata O, Shiono M, et al. Extracorporeal shock wave therapy for resistant stress fracture in athletes: a report of 5 cases. Am J Sports Med 2007;35(7): 1188–92.
70. Albisetti W, Perugia D, De Bartolomeo O, et al. Stress fractures of the base of the metatarsal bones in young trainee ballet dancers. Int Orthop 2010;34(1):51–5.
71. Lüthje P, Nurmi-Lüthje I. Non-union of the clavicle and delayed union of the proximal fifth metatarsal treated with low-intensity pulsed ultrasound in two soccer players. J Sports Med Phys Fitness 2006;46(3):476–80.
72. Shindle MK, Endo Y, Warren RF, et al. Stress fractures about the tibia, foot, and ankle. J Am Acad Orthop Surg 2012;20(3):167–76.
73. Kesani AK, Gandhi A, Lin SS. Electrical bone stimulation devices in foot and ankle surgery: types of devices, scientific basis, and clinical indications for their use. Foot Ankle Int 2006;27(2):148–56.
74. Holmes GB Jr. Treatment of delayed unions and nonunions of the proximal fifth metatarsal with pulsed electromagnetic fields. Foot Ankle Int 1994;15(10):552–6.
75. Benazzo F, Mosconi M, Beccarisi G, et al. Use of capacitive coupled electric fields in stress fractures in athletes. Clin Orthop Relat Res 1995;(310):145–9.
76. Hulkko A, Orava S, Nikula P. Stress fracture of the fifth metatarsal in athletes. Ann Chir Gynaecol 1985;74(5):233–8.
77. Sarimo J, Rantanen J, Orava S, et al. Tension-band wiring for fractures of the fifth metatarsal located in the junction of the proximal metaphysis and diaphysis. Am J Sports Med 2006;34(3):476–80.
78. Khan WS, Agarwal M, Warren-Smith C. Management of fractures of the base of the fifth metatarsals distal to the tuberosity. Foot 2005;15:141–5.
79. Portland G, Kelikian A, Kodros S. Acute surgical management of Jones' fractures. Foot Ankle Int 2003;24(11):829–33.
80. Hens J, Martens M. Surgical treatment of Jones fractures. Arch Orthop Trauma Surg 1990;109(5):277–9.
81. Habbu RA, Marsh RS, Anderson JG, et al. Closed intramedullary screw fixation for nonunion of fifth metatarsal Jones fracture. Foot Ankle Int 2011;32(6): 603–8.
82. Porter DA, Rund AM, Dobslaw R, et al. Comparison of 4.5- and 5.5-mm cannulated stainless steel screws for fifth metatarsal Jones fracture fixation. Foot Ankle Int 2009;30(1):27–33.

Tibialis Posterior Tendon and Deltoid and Spring Ligament Injuries in the Elite Athlete

William John Ribbans, PhD, FRCSOrth, FFSEM(UK)[a],*,
Ajit Garde, FRCSOrth[b]

KEYWORDS

- Tibialis posterior tendon • Deltoid ligament • Spring ligament • Elite athletes

KEY POINTS

- Isolated deltoid ligament injuries account for no more than 3% to 4% of all ankle ligament injuries.
- Acute isolated deltoid ligament injuries promptly diagnosed can usually be treated conservatively.
- Untreated acute tears of the spring ligament in the athlete can lead to progressive deformity similar to tibialis posterior dysfunction.
- There is little place for conservative treatment of complete acute spring ligament tears in the elite athlete; minor tears with no deformity may be considered for cast immobilization.
- For tibialis tendon problems, most insertional and early tendon abnormalities can be treated conservatively with attention to underlying biomechanical and technical deficits.
- Surgical interventions should only be considered after an adequate period of assessment and conservative treatment. In the absence of significant disability, simple synovectomy and decompression may suffice.

INTRODUCTION

Injuries to the medial side of the ankle and foot in the athlete can involve several different structures, abnormalities, and grades of injury. The tibialis posterior tendon (TPT) and the spring and deltoid ligament complexes combine to provide dynamic and passive stabilization on the medial side of the ankle and hindfoot.

Articles dealing with the full spectrum of pathology in relation to these structures abound. This article does not cover those abnormalities incompatible with elite sport (eg, Grade III and IV tibialis posterior dysfunction[1] and chronic ligament instability)

[a] The University of Northampton, School of Health, Park Campus, Northampton NN2 7AL, UK; [b] Northampton General Hospital, Northampton NN1 5BD, UK
* Corresponding author. The County Clinic, 57 Billing Road, Northampton NN1 5DB, UK.
E-mail address: billribbs@uk-doctors.co.uk

Foot Ankle Clin N Am 18 (2013) 255–291
http://dx.doi.org/10.1016/j.fcl.2013.02.006
1083-7515/13/$ – see front matter © 2013 Elsevier Inc. All rights reserved.

foot.theclinics.com

that create significant degenerative changes. Here the following conditions are reviewed:

Spring Ligament
- Isolated spring ligament injury
- Spring ligament involvement in tibialis posterior insufficiency

Deltoid Ligament Complex
- Acute isolated injury of the deltoid ligament
- Deltoid ligament involvement in ankle fractures
- Combined injury to the lateral and medial ligamentous complexes of the ankle
- Combined injury to the syndesmotic and medial ligamentous complexes of the ankle
- Chronic instability of the deltoid ligament
- Medial impingement of the ankle
- Osseous abnormalities at the tip of the medial malleolus

Tibialis Posterior Tendon
- Stage I and II disease of the TPT
- TPT tears
- TPT acute rupture
- TPT dislocation
- TPT lacerations
- Accessory navicular problems

Some of these injuries will involve acute injuries to previously healthy structures, but many will have developed insidiously with underlying chronic pathologic conditions. It behooves the clinician to be aware of new treatment strategies and the level of accompanying scientific evidence while acknowledging that more traditional management applied to nonathletic patients is still likely to be appropriate in the elite setting. In dealing with damage to these structures, the test for the clinician is in providing effective treatment with the goal of retaining the athlete's elite status, something that is not always achievable.

SPRING LIGAMENT
Anatomy

At Chopart's level the foot contains a relatively stable, rigid lateral column, including the calcaneocuboid joint, and a more flexible medial column containing the talocalcaneonavicular joint.

The talocalcaneonavicular joint comprises an articulation between:

- Talar head
- Acetabulum pedis, involving the anterior and middle articular facets of the calcaneum, the talar articular surface of the navicular, and the spring ligament. The term acetabulum pedis was first described by Sarrafian[2]

The talocalcaneonavicular joint is supported by the talonavicular ligament and the spring ligament, with additional support from the tibionavicular part of the deltoid ligament. The extent and number of components of the spring ligament varies in different publications. It is best considered as comprising the following (**Fig. 1**)[3]:

- Superomedial calcaneonavicular ligament (SMCNL):
  - The most medial and largest of the 3 ligaments. It is triangular and hammock-shaped. It originates from the entire anterior margin of the middle facet of the subtalar joint. It runs distally alongside the medial tubercle of the navicular, without attaching to it, before finally inserting onto the superior part of the medial side of the navicular articular margin.
- Inferoplantar longitudinal calcaneonavicular ligament (ICNL):
  - The most lateral of the 3 components. It is short and broad. It arises from between the anterior and middle facets of the subtalar joint and passes to the lateral navicular beak.
- Third (medioplantar oblique) calcaneonavicular ligament:
  - The third ligament was first described by Taniguchi and colleagues.[4] It lies between the other 2 ligaments. It is striplike and starts from between the anterior and middle facets of the subtalar joint medial to the inferoplantar ligament. It attaches to the navicular tuberosity.

The articular surface of the spring ligament supports the talar head along with the TPT, which runs inferior to the spring ligament. This ligament surface, principally on the deep surface of the SMCNL, is covered with articular fibrocartilage, allowing it to form an articulation with the inferior aspect of the talus; this is termed the spring ligament fibrocartilaginous complex.

The SMCNL is intimately connected to both the TPT and the superficial component of the deltoid ligament via the latter's tibiospring ligament component, allowing the complexes to interact to provide medial stability for the ankle and hindfoot.

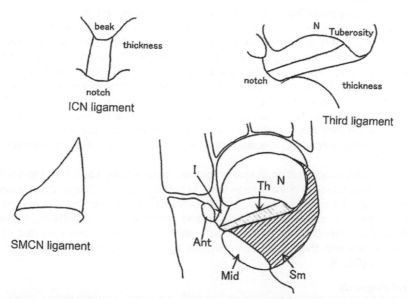

Fig. 1. The spring ligament and the acetabulum pedis. Ant, anterior facet of os calcis; I, ICN ligaments; Mid, middle facet of os calcis; N, navicular; Sm, SMCN ligament; Th, Third ligament. (*Adapted from* Taniguchi A, Tanaka Y, Takakura Y, et al. Anatomy of the spring ligament. J Bone Joint Surg Am 2003;85:2177; with permission.)

Biomechanics

The spring ligament helps maintain arch height and stability, and resists forefoot abduction.

Kitaoka and colleagues[5] considered several ligaments to be important in the maintenance of arch height: plantar fascia; long and short plantar ligaments; spring ligament; medial talocalcaneal ligament; talocalcaneal interosseous ligament; and the tibionavicular part of the deltoid ligament. The spring ligament was considered to be less important than others, based on most parameters tested. Iaquinto and Wayne,[6] using a computational model, attributed only 8% of the total ligament contribution to arch stability to the spring ligament, compared with 79.5% to the plantar fascia.

Conversely, Hollinshead[7] regarded the spring ligament as important in maintaining medial arch stability. Davis and colleagues[8] considered the complex important as a sling for the talar head. The SMCNL has properties suggestive of a significant load-bearing function, whereas the ICNL has more of a pure tensile load function. Jennings and Christensen[9] sectioned the spring ligament in cadaveric studies and concluded that division of the spring ligament complex produced instability, uncompensated for by active tibialis posterior contraction, and considered it the main stabilizer of the arch during midstance.

Deland[10] found that sectioning of the spring ligament alone in a cadaveric model failed to produce immediate major deformity. However, subsequent cyclical loading of the foot, deprived of an intact spring ligament, produces deformity.

Injury

Spring ligament injuries seen at surgery for TPT deficiency occur most commonly in the SMCNL.[10,11] Although ICNL injuries can occur (**Fig. 5**),[10] they are not so easily observed because of their position and, probably in isolation, are not so critical for foot mechanics.

Most spring ligament injuries occur in conjunction with TPT dysfunction. Gazdag and Cracchiolo[11] reported tears in the SMCNL in 82% of patients. Balen and Helms[12] found that 92% of patients with TPT dysfunction had damage to the SMCNL on magnetic resonance imaging (MRI). Isolated injuries to the spring ligament have been occasionally reported in the literature, but not with great frequency.[10,13–17] Whereas the SMCNL is most commonly implicated in isolated injuries, a complete rupture of the spring ligament complex can occur, for instance in association with talonavicular dislocations.[18] During explosive athletic events, such as triple jumping,[13] the significant strain placed on the spring ligament is capable of producing repetitive microtrauma and degeneration or, on occasions, sudden catastrophic failure.

The orientation and position of spring ligament tears varies. Most MRI reports indicate gapping suggestive of transverse tears in the SMCNL.[19,20] Surgical observations frequently report transverse injury.[13,21] Hintermann[22] observed that the lesions are usually larger than expected, often distal and involving several patterns, including longitudinal L-shaped tears. Hintermann[21] also noted combination injuries of the spring ligament with the deltoid tibionavicular ligament and in association with TPT lengthening (**Fig. 5**).

Clinical diagnosis

In acute situations, the athlete will identify the occasion and mechanism of injury. Hintermann[22] reports that acute injury is usually caused by a pronation force. Early examination may reveal medial swelling and bruising. Tenderness will be located on the medial and plantar aspects of the foot.

Others may present with a more insidious onset suggesting progressive weakening of the ligament subjected to high stresses, often in association with excessive body weight.[16] Progressively, the patient may note increasing hindfoot valgus deformity, forefoot abduction of the forefoot, and collapse of the medial arch.

In association with TPT dysfunction, the disability demonstrated will be dominated by the malfunctioning tendon. In cases of isolated injury, the patient will retain full (Grade 5) tibialis posterior strength, and Hintermann[21,22] has demonstrated how tendon activation corrects the medial arch height (**Fig. 2**).

The case report by Borton and Saxby[13] was unable to undertake repetitive single heel raises and was unable to invert the heel. Tryfonidis and colleagues[16] described all 9 patients with isolated spring ligament injuries retaining the ability to single-stance tiptoe with correction of the medial arch height, but without correction of the heel valgus translation and persistent forefoot abduction.

Classification
Gazdag and Cracchiolo[11] provided a classification of spring ligament injuries based on perioperative observations of patients undergoing reconstruction for TPT insufficiency who were observed to have simultaneous ligament injuries (**Table 1**). Hintermann[21] includes spring ligament injury in conjunction with deltoid tibionavicular ligament injury as the Type III (distal) lesion in his classification of medial ankle instability.

Imaging
Imaging for a suspected spring ligament injury commences with plain radiography. Weight-bearing anteroposterior (AP) and lateral views of the foot and ankle combined with oblique foot images and Cobey views[23] for hindfoot alignment give a comprehensive assessment for alignment, deformity, subtle avulsion injuries, and early degenerative changes. Plain radiography in the chronic situation, especially in relation to TPT dysfunction, may show changes commonly associated with the latter, particularly midfoot sag, hindfoot valgus, and midfoot abduction.

Further imaging of the spring ligament requires the use of MRI and/or ultrasonography. MRI is more reliable for SMCNL, which is seen well on routine axial and coronal views. The inferior check ligament (ICL), which is thinner and smaller, is less easily visualized, although Rule and colleagues[24] described specific oblique, sagittal, and axial imaging sequences to better image this portion. Lack of homogeneity of MRI signal in the proximal ICL is common and should not be interpreted as necessarily indicating abnormality.[20]

Acute SMCNL injuries are associated with evidence of fresh injury: soft-tissue and osseous edema, hematoma formation in the early stages, and gapping of the ligament (**Fig. 3**).

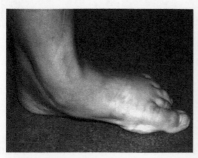
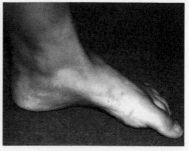

Fig. 2. Patient with spring ligament injury activating tibialis posterior tendon to restore normal medial arch. (*Courtesy of* Professor Beat Hintermann, Orthopaedic Clinic, Kantonsspital, CH-4410 Liestal, Switzerland.)

Table 1		
Classification by Gazdag and Cracchiolo (1997)		
Grade	Observation	Number (N = 18)
1	Longitudinal tear	7
2	Laxity without obvious tear	7
3	Complete rupture	4

Data from Gazdag AR, Cracchiolo A. Rupture of the posterior tibial tendon. Evaluation of injury of the spring ligament and clinical assessment of tendon transfer and ligament repair. J Bone Joint Surg Am 1997;79(5):675–81.

Chronic injuries occur usually in conjunction with TPT tendinopathy. Abnormalities of the SMCNL on MRI evaluation were reported by Yao and colleagues[19] as having 54% to 77% sensitivity and 100% specificity in detecting abnormality. Rather than show significant thinning, Yao and coleagues[19] and Toye and colleagues[20] described SMCNL thickening (usually >5 mm[19]). In addition, Toye and colleagues[20] described other features such as increased signal on T2-weighted images, full-thickness gapping, and ligament waviness. Because of MRI sensitivity, some of these abnormal features on imaging of the SMCNL were regarded as normal at surgery. It should be noted that normal controls may show spring ligament abnormalities (17%–28%).[19,20]

Spring ligament injuries can be diagnosed by experienced radiologists using ultrasonography.[16] Harish and colleagues[25] confirmed that the SMCNL was readily identified and its thickness quantifiable in both cadaveric and asymptomatic individuals. A 94% concordance between ultrasonography and MRI in the diagnosis of spring ligament injuries, mostly in association with TPT abnormality, has been recorded.[26] In addition, ultrasonography confirms any concomitant TPT abnormality.

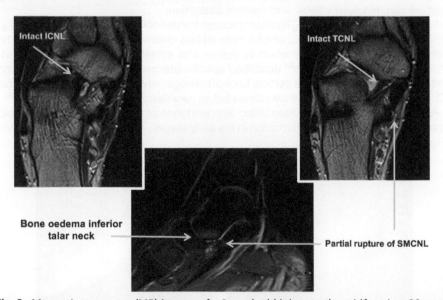

Intact ICNL

Intact TCNL

Bone oedema inferior talar neck

Partial rupture of SMCNL

Fig. 3. Magnetic resonance (MR) images of a 3-week old injury to the midfoot in a 20-year-old footballer, demonstrating an acute partial rupture of the superomedial calcaneonavicular ligament, and intact inferoplantar longitudinal calcaneonavicular ligament and third calcaneonavicular ligament.

Treatment: Conservative

There is little place for conservative treatment of acute complete tears or chronic injury with progressive deformity in elite athletes. For acute partial injury, it is reasonable to place the leg in a non–weight-bearing cast for up to 6 weeks, after which progressive rehabilitation should be instituted. Return to high-impact sport should not be allowed until all biomechanical issues have been rectified, full strength restored, and suitable orthotic support agreed. Tryfonidis and colleagues[16] treated 6 of 9 patients conservatively with orthotics for an acute partial injury to the SMCNL with surrounding soft-tissue edema and bleeding, but no clinical or imaging deformity.

Treatment: Surgical

The choice of a particular surgical option for a torn spring ligament depends on whether it is being repaired or reconstructed as part of a more extensive procedure to correct a planovalgus deformity, secondary to TPT dysfunction, or as an isolated injury. Most experience has been gained in the former, and the value of a specific repair for a damaged spring ligament in such circumstances remains undetermined. Mann[27] reported no difference in outcomes between 49 patients receiving no spring ligament repair and 26 repaired during TPT reconstruction. However, the exact technique was not reported. A 2002 review of surgical practice revealed that 53% of orthopedic surgeons repair the SMCNL as part of routine reconstruction of an adult-acquired planovalgus foot.[28]

Considerations for surgery to the spring ligament itself need to include the following issues.

- Is the tear and tissue quality such that repair is possible and, if so, which technique should be used?
- If the ligament is not suitable for repair, some form of reconstruction is required. The choices include various forms of autografts, allografts, or synthetic material. Recommendations are significantly limited, as published series are small and several potential techniques have been undertaken on cadaveric tissue only.
- Do any other structures require repair or reconstruction (eg, TPT, deltoid ligament)?
- Does the repair/reconstruction require protection from additional procedures such as hindfoot osteotomies?

Direct repair is possible. Gazdag and Cracchiolo[11] repaired longitudinal tears, and Tryfonidis and colleagues[16] undertook an isolated repair in one of their series. Borton and Saxby[13] repaired a case 6 months after injury using a plication or "vest over pants" technique. Hintermann[21] also described direct suturing. Goldner and colleagues[29] reconstructed the ligament in 6 patients by ligament advancement and plication.

However, only 1 of these cases[16] did not have additional reinforcement or protection. Three patients had the repaired spring ligament reinforced with a flexor digitorum longus (FDL) transfer,[13,16] with 1 undergoing an additional medializing calcaneal osteotomy.[16] Goldner and colleagues[29] reinforced the repair with the tendon graft used to reconstruct the incompetent posterior tibial tendon (PTT).

Seventeen of 18 patients in the series of Gazdag and Cracchiolo[11] had FDL transfers to reconstruct the TPT. In addition, 6 had the repaired spring ligament reinforced by a modification of the Cobb repair using half of a longitudinally split tibialis anterior tendon, and another 4 were reinforced using the distal TPT stump.

Deland and colleagues[30] used an in vitro model to test the suitability of the anterior deltoid for reconstruction but were not successful clinically[10] and, similarly, Gazdag and Cracchiolo[11] explored 3 of their patients with a view to using the superficial fibers of the deltoid for reinforcement, but deemed the tissue inadequate.

Future surgical options might include the use of allografts, for instance Achilles tendon allograft, which has been tested in cadaveric specimens,[31] or synthetic materials such as Artelon, a polycaprolactone-based polyurethane urea, which acts as a scaffold for host tissue ingrowth, particularly type I collagen, to reconstruct a torn or incompetent spring ligament (**Fig. 4**).

Choi and colleagues[32] and Thordarson and colleagues[31] described spring ligament reconstruction using the peroneus longus (PL) in cadavers with different tunnels and fixation techniques. The PL is divided laterally proximal to the lateral malleolus and delivered through a medial incision, retaining its attachment to the base of the first metatarsal. One concern over harvesting the PL is the loss of its plantarflexion function on the first ray. However, as the tendon is sutured under tension in its new ligamentous role, it is presumed that its plantarflexion action is retained. Although Deland[10] described one patient who had undergone a reconstruction using PL, Williams and colleagues[33] described a series of 14 feet (13 patients) that underwent spring ligament reconstruction using a PL autograft. However, the technique was only used in patients who had persistent forefoot abduction or talonavicular sag after hindfoot osteotomies, including lateral column lengthening.

The requirement for further osseous procedures to protect any ligament repair or reconstruction has been described. Otis and colleagues[34] produced cadaver evidence that medial displacement osteotomies of the calcaneum unload the spring ligament. Lateral column lengthening, as used by Williams and colleagues,[33] reduces talonavicular abduction and SMCNL tension.

Hintermann[22] advises additional repair of concomitant deltoid ligament injuries. For degenerative joint change or fixed deformities, he advocated consideration of arthrodesis.

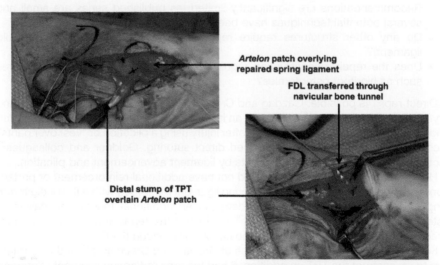

Artelon patch overlying repaired spring ligament

FDL transferred through navicular bone tunnel

Distal stump of TPT overlain *Artelon* patch

Fig. 4. Reconstruction of degenerate spring ligament. The patient had a Stage II tibialis posterior tendon with an incompetent tibialis posterior tendon (TPT), symptomatic os naviculare, and torn spring ligament. The medial reconstruction involved excision of the os naviculare, spring ligament reconstruction with an Artelon patch overlaid with the distal TPT, and a flexor digitorum longus transfer.

The results of surgery are difficult to summarize, with so many techniques and small numbers in published series. Gazdag and Cracchiolo[11] reported that 78% had excellent results with a follow-up between 24 and 40 months. Williams and colleagues[33] reported an average increase in American Orthopaedic Foot and Ankle Society score from 43 to 90 at an average follow-up of 8.9 years.

Learning points for spring ligament injuries in elite sport

- Isolated spring ligament injuries have been reported in sport but are rare.
- The deforming force is usually pronation, and most commonly involves the SMCNL portion.
- Clinical features mimic many of those of tibialis posterior dysfunction, and commonly occur together.
- However, an intact and functioning TPT on examination and imaging should raise the suspicion of spring ligament injury. Confirmatory clinical signs include deformity correction from active tibialis posterior contraction.
- MRI is the most reliable imaging modality. On imaging soft-tissue and osseous edema, hematoma formation and ligament gapping are seen in the acute stages on MRI.
- Untreated acute tears in the athlete can lead to progressive deformity similar to tibialis posterior dysfunction.
- There is little place for conservative treatment of complete acute tears in the elite athlete; minor tears with no deformity may be considered for cast immobilization.
- A preferred technique for surgical repair/reconstruction has not been established because of the paucity of published information. However, simple repair is unlikely to be sufficient even in an elite athlete.

DELTOID LIGAMENT
Anatomy

The deltoid ligament consists of superficial and deep layers. The number of individual components and assignment to each layer is a matter of debate. Sarrafian[35] noted 13 different descriptions of the ligament's anatomy since 1822.

The superficial layer according to Milner and Soames[36] consists of 4 components based on the insertion of the various parts. The origin for each component is from the anterior colliculus of the medial malleolus. Combined they form a continuous triangular ligament, which spans both the ankle joint and subtalar joint (except the tibiotalar). It is acknowledged that not all are constant.

- Tibiospring: attaches to the SMCNL part of the spring ligament, allowing an interplay between the 2 ligament complexes to support the medial side of the ankle
- Tibionavicular: attaches to the dorsomedial surface of the navicular
- Tibiocalcaneal: descends vertically to the sustenaculum tali
- Tibiotalar: attaches to the medial talar tubercle

The deep layer spans the ankle joint only. It is shorter and thicker than, and is distinct from, the superficial layer. Milner and Soames[36] described 2 layers:

- The deep anterior tibiotalar layer arises from the anterior colliculus. It is short and small, and attaches to the medial side of the talus immediately distal to the articular surface.
- The deep posterior tibiotalar layer is the strongest part of the whole medial collateral ligament complex. Arising from the intercollicular groove and posterior colliculus, this cone-shaped structure inserts into the medial talus.

Other investigators recognize only 2 superficial components, placing the superficial tibiotalar component as part of the deep layer and recategorizing the tibionavicular layer as no more than a thickening of the anteromedial capsule.[37] The same investigators recognized the confusion in previously published anatomic articles and the lack of descriptive consistency in articles on surgical technique. Boss and Hintermann[37] surmised that the superficial layer consists of only those ligaments spanning 2 joints (tibiospring and tibiocalcaneal) together with the capsular thickening, forming the tibionavicular and the 2 deep and 1 superficial (renamed intermediate) tibiotalar ligaments that together comprise the deep layer spanning only the ankle joint.

Function

The function and activity of various components of the deltoid ligament have not been consistently reported. The deltoid ligament resists abduction of the talus within the ankle mortise.[38] Harper[39] stated that the superficial and deep components were equally effective in resisting talar eversion, with the tibiocalcaneal part being the strongest component. The deep components of the deltoid complex resist lateral displacement of the talus. Rasmussen and colleagues[40] reported that the superficial layer is stronger in limiting external rotation and that the deep layer can rupture in external rotation without the superficial component failing. However, in supination–external rotation (Weber type B) and pronation–external rotation (Weber type C) fractures, Michelson and colleagues[41,42] reported the key role of the deep deltoid component.

The deltoid ligament requires considerable force to be disrupted. The deep component of the complex is stronger than the lateral ligaments under load[43] but weaker than the posterior tibiofibular component of the syndesmosis.[44] When the posterior tibiotalar ligament fails, it usually occurs distally and intrasubstance.[44]

Injury

Deltoid ligament injuries should be considered as acute or chronic.
Acute injuries can be further subdivided:

- Isolated deltoid injuries
- In association with ankle fractures
- Combination ligament injuries
  - With lateral collateral ligament injuries
  - With syndesmotic ligament injuries
  - With spring ligament injuries

Chronic injuries can be considered as:

- Chronic sequelae of acute injuries
- Combined with TPT insufficiency and/or insidious spring ligament damage

Classification

There have been few attempts to provide comprehensive classification systems for medial ligament injuries. Hintermann's classification[21] is based on the anatomic location of the injury (**Fig. 5**, **Table 2**):

Acute injury

Isolated injury Isolated deltoid ligament injuries are relatively rare. An incidence of 3% to 4%[45,46] in all ankle sprains has been reported. Frequently the patient will describe an eversion, external rotation, or abduction mechanism. Isolated deltoid ligament injuries have been reported in athletes.[47,48] However, Harper[49] reported that all 42 patients with complete deltoid ligament ruptures were associated with other injuries.

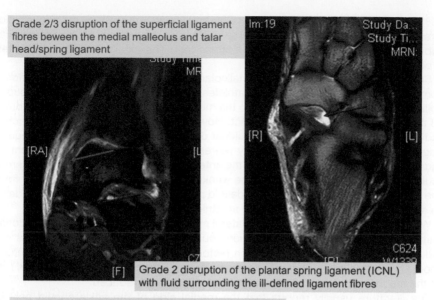

Grade 2/3 disruption of the superficial ligament fibres beween the medial malleolus and talar head/spring ligament

Grade 2 disruption of the plantar spring ligament (ICNL) with fluid surrounding the ill-defined ligament fibres

Coronal PD FSE and T2 Fat Sat anterior talar dome

Fig. 5. MRI coronal and axial images of combined injury to the superficial deltoid and the ICNL component of the spring ligament.

Deltoid ligament injury in ankle fractures Deltoid injuries occur commonly in relation to fractures, for example supination–external rotation, pronation-abduction, and pronation–external rotation injuries.[49–52]

Establishing the stability in these fractures is important in determining prognosis and planning treatment. In supination–external rotation fractures (Weber type B) only 2.8% of stable fractures had arthritis at an average of 18 years' follow-up. In nonoperated unstable fractures, 65.5% developed osteoarthritis at a mean of 6.8 years, a figure reduced to 20.9% (mean 5.5 years) with surgery.[53]

Medial swelling, tenderness, and bruising are sought in such injuries. Review of the plain radiographs looks for evidence of injury to the medial ligamentous structures, for example, widening of the medial clear space (normally 2–4 mm) on mortise views. However, none of these parameters are certain predictors of deep deltoid ligament damage.[54] With preoperative radiographs showing a normal medial clear space in supination-external type fractures, De Angelis and colleagues[55] reported that only

Table 2			
Hintermann's classification of deltoid ligament injuries (2003)			
Lesion Type	Location	Ligaments Involved	Incidence (%)
I	Proximal tear or avulsion	Tibionavicular; tibiospring	72
II	Intermediate: Deep component remains attached distally; superficial component remains attached proximally	Tibionavicular; tibiospring	9
III	Distal = most common	Tibionavicular; spring (see **Fig. 5**)	19

Data from Hintermann B. Medial ankle instability. Foot Ankle Clin 2003;8(4):723–38.

25% of patients with medial tenderness had a subsequent positive external rotation stress mortise radiograph test. Likewise, 25% of patients with no tenderness had subsequent instability on performing a stress test. The external rotation stress test is considered the gold standard.[54]

Satisfactory reduction of a medial malleolar fracture does not assure restoration of competence of the deltoid ligament in athletes. Tornetta[52] demonstrated that in supracollicular fractures (proximal injuries to the medial malleolus with a minimum width of 28 mm), the deltoid ligament was intact. However, more distal injuries, with fracture widths of less than 17 mm, risked residual deltoid incompetence despite adequate fragment fixation. Such an injury may represent a combined osseous-ligamentous injury. The fracture fragment contains the anterior colliculus and some of the intercollicular groove carrying the origin of the weaker superficial ligament. The injury force line exits posteriorly through the deep deltoid portion. This injury should be considered as a source of long-term weakness in an athlete and, if confirmed, repaired.

With an intact medial malleolus the lateral malleolus fracture is reduced, and confirmation of satisfactory mortise reduction sought by fluoroscopy. If the fibula is well reduced and the mortise configuration restored, the medial ligamentous structures should heal adequately. Harper[49] demonstrated no chronic medial instability as long as the medial joint space and lateral malleolus were well reduced.

The literature usually reports that the medial side of the ankle should only be explored if there is a block to reduction indicating imbrication of torn deltoid ligament fibers into the joint. However, in the case of elite athletes a low threshold should be held for surgical inspection of the medial structures to minimize the risk of later subtle instability symptoms. A persistent increase in the medial clear space (>3 mm) was reported by Maynou and colleagues[56] to require surgical exploration. Early surgical repair in the presence of extensive swelling and bleeding is not always technically easy, and the deep deltoid component is relatively short in length.

Combined injury to the lateral and medial ligamentous complexes of the ankle Many athletes with significant lateral ligament injury demonstrate medial ligament abnormality on imaging, even in the absence of symptoms.

MRI of patients requiring lateral ligament reconstruction for instability demonstrated a high concomitant prevalence of medial ligament injury even though the patients were asymptomatic with regard to medial pain or instability.[57] The investigators found that 72% had MRI evidence of deltoid ligament injury (23% superficial fibers only; 6% deep fibers only; 43% combined). Thus 32% of patients with evidence of superficial deltoid injury had an intact deep component. Superficial deltoid ligament injury most commonly occurred proximally at its origin. All of the patients in this series had damage to the anterior talofibular ligament laterally, with either or both the calcaneofibular ligament and posterior talofibular ligament involved. Hintermann and colleagues[58] found that 40% of patients with a combination of chronic ankle instability and medial and lateral ankle pain had deltoid injury.

In chronic rotational instability, caused by a combination of medial and lateral ligament injury, Buchhorn and colleagues[59] found that the tibiocalcaneal component of the deltoid complex was most commonly involved on the medial side, with a minority of patients sustaining additionally an avulsion of the origin of the deep anterior tibiotalar component. This combination injury requires repair on both sides of the ankle.

Combined injury to the syndesmosis and medial ligamentous complexes of the ankle High ankle sprains cause injury to the syndesmotic complex and account for about 10% of ankle sprains, with a range in the literature from 1% to 18%.[46,60,61] Although the mechanism of injury is unlikely to be identical in all cases, external rotation of a dorsiflexed ankle is a common description. There is a variety of patterns and combinations of ligament injuries, but involvement of the deltoid ligament is common. Evaluation of the injury usually concentrates on the severity of injury to the syndesmotic complex and the development of a diastasis, however subtle. Attention should be paid to the presence of medial tenderness and the appearance of the deltoid complex on imaging. In cases requiring surgical intervention, management of the syndesmostic injury usually will effect satisfactory reduction, but an inability to reduce the mortise in unstable cases should raise suspicions of an infolded torn deltoid ligament.

Chronic injury
Acute injuries, either isolated or combined with other ligament or osseous injuries, may cause chronic symptoms, alignment alterations, and feelings of instability if the diagnosis is not made and/or the injury is undertreated.

Chronic deltoid insufficiency problems are often associated with TPT dysfunction; indeed the 2 are intimately related in maintenance of medial stability, and damage to one can lead to overload and failure of the other.[62] In addition, they may occur in combination with spring ligament injuries, and are classified by Hintermann[21] as a Type III lesion.

Clinical features The patient often reports a feeling of a "pop" on the medial side of the ankle, which is usually followed by pain and swelling. Implicated sports include soccer, American football, basketball, long jump and triple jump, and dancing. The patient complains of instability or giving way on the medial side.

In conjunction with instability, Hintermann and colleagues[63] reported medial gutter pain (100%), pain associated with the TPT (27%), and pain on the anterior border of the lateral malleolus (25%).

On weight bearing, the affected foot is held in hindfoot valgus and pronation, which becomes more pronounced with chronicity. However, because the TPT is usually intact and functioning, the patient can correct the deformity by actively contracting this muscle, which helps distinguish the isolated deltoid ligament injury from combination abnormality with the tendon. Similarly, the intact tibialis posterior is activated on tiptoe and corrects the valgus hindfoot and foot pronation position.[21]

Examination should seek evidence of additional osseous injury, and lateral and syndesmotic ligament involvement.

Clinical stress testing is best undertaken with the leg dependent and the patient sitting at the end of the examination couch. Both ankles are compared on valgus, varus, external rotation, and anterior drawer testing.

Imaging of the deltoid ligament complex Radiographs of the ankle and hindfoot will exclude injuries to the lateral malleolus, and more subtle osseous injuries to the medial side of the ankle may be noted, including avulsion fractures of the talus.[64] With fractures and/or syndesmotic injuries, evidence of widening of the medial clear space is sought. In isolated deltoid ruptures, the medial clear space cannot widen because the intact lateral malleolus will hold the talus in position.

For more chronic injuries, the hindfoot may adopt a valgus deformity with talar tilt within the mortise noted on weight-bearing ankle AP radiographs. Assessment of alignment can be gained from hindfoot[23] or long-axial views.[65]

Stress radiography for isolated deltoid injuries and for those in association with fractures, combined lateral-medial instability, or syndesmotic injuries can be used to corroborate clinical examination findings. Examination of the ankle with external rotation stresses applied is undertaken. Gravity stress tests in cases of supination-external rotation fractures are reported as being equally accurate.[66] Hintermann and colleagues[63] reported stress testing as not useful in the evaluation of chronic cases.

Historically, arthrography was used to assess both lateral and medial collateral ligament ankle injury. With other modalities available, it is rarely used now.

Ultrasonography has been used to evaluate the competency of the deltoid ligament in cases of supination–external rotation fractures.[67,68] Both sensitivity and specificity reached 100%, and helped guide management in these groups in distinguishing between stable and unstable fractures.

Better quality of MRI and improved understanding of the deltoid ligament anatomy allows improved resolution of abnormalities of this complex and identification of the individual components (**Figs. 5** and **6**).[69]

The only indication for CT in investigating deltoid ligament abnormality is for the evaluation of associated avulsion injuries and osseous abnormalities, and the exclusion of a talocalcaneal coalition.

Treatment

Conservative treatment

Acute surgical repair is rarely required for isolated deltoid ligament injuries. Prompt diagnosis allows the ankle to be rested and initially protected. Once the acute swelling and pain has subsided, a functional rehabilitation program can be introduced. The outcome is usually good or excellent.

For combination injuries, the decision to treat conservatively will usually depend on the assessment of the accompanying fracture, syndesmotic injury, or lateral ligament injury.

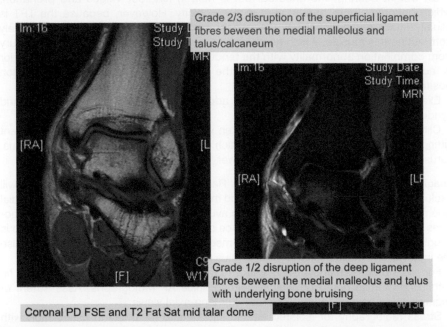

Grade 2/3 disruption of the superficial ligament fibres beween the medial malleolus and talus/calcaneum

Grade 1/2 disruption of the deep ligament fibres beween the medial malleolus and talus with underlying bone bruising

Coronal PD FSE and T2 Fat Sat mid talar dome

Fig. 6. MR images of deltoid ligament anatomy. Coronal proton-density fast spin-echo and T2-weighted fat-saturated images of the mid talar dome.

In chronic cases, conservative treatment might be followed in certain patient groups, but it is unlikely to be successful in the elite athlete. Taping, bracing, and orthotics combined with a strengthening and proprioceptive program can be undertaken as an initial trial, but continuing pain and instability are indications for surgical intervention.

Surgery
In acute cases involving fractures or syndesmotic injuries, the indications and principles of surgical management of the deltoid component have already been discussed.
Planning for surgery to the deltoid ligament includes the following decisions:

- Is an initial ankle arthroscopy going to aid management of the problem?
- How is the deltoid ligament going to be exposed?
- Can the ligament be repaired and, if so, what equipment is needed to achieve a satisfactory outcome?
- If the ligament needs reconstructing, what techniques can be used?
- What other structures need inspecting?
- Are any additional osseous procedures required?

Ankle arthroscopy Hintermann[21] encouraged the use of ankle arthroscopy before actual deltoid ligament surgery. As in cases of lateral ligament instability, it allows for inspection of the intra-articular ankle structures and management of any identified abnormality. Hintermann[21] graded the stability of the ankle during arthroscopy as stable, when the tibiotalar joint cannot be opened by more than 2 mm; moderately unstable, with the ankle joint opening up to 5 mm; and severely unstable, when the talus is moved easily out of the mortise.

Surgical approach to the deltoid ligament A gently curving incision from the medial malleolus to the medial part of the talonavicular joint is made. Following division of the overlying laciniate ligament, the anterior tibionavicular part of the superficial component of the deltoid ligament is inspected. The TPT sheath is opened longitudinally and the tendon inspected. TPT retraction allows visualization of the superficial layer of the deltoid ligament and the SMCNL component of the spring ligament.

Surgical repair or reconstruction of the deltoid ligament Surgery to the deltoid ligament itself depends on the site and extent of the lesion and is aided by preoperative planning. Plain radiography and/or CT may have identified avulsion injuries or the presence of accessory ossicles such as the os tibiale. MRI can identify whether the superficial, deep, or both components are involved and if the injuries are proximal, midsubstance, or distal, which can differ in the superficial and deep components.

At the very least, the ligament will require repair or reattachment. Suitable suture material and anchors should be available. Take time in inspecting the ligament. For acute injuries, accompanied by lateral ligamentous or osseous damage, the site of damage is usually clear, allowing either ligament repair or reattachment.

A full tear to 1 or more parts of the superficial component allows gentle mobilization and inspection of the deep fibers at the level of the injury. If the superficial component appears intact it can be carefully divided transversely, avoiding unnecessary injury to the deep component, and the 2 parts reflected superiorly and inferiorly.

Hintermann and colleagues[63] reported prospectively a group of 52 patients whose damaged, unstable deltoid ligaments were suitable for repair, and Raikin and Myerson[64] recorded that the tissue, even in chronic cases, was usually adequate for reconstruction.

Hintermann and colleagues[62] describe surgical techniques for the direct repair of both acute and chronic injuries, different levels, and different components. The principles for each, however, include careful dissection and identification of the lesions, secure fixation to bone with anchors, and correct tensioning.

If the tissues are inadequate for a stable repair, alternatives have been described:

- Free autografts in the form of a hamstring tendon, plantaris tendon, or FDL tendon[70,71]
- Attached autografts such as a split TPT or PL[62,72,73]
- Allografts[47,62,74–77]

Cadaver studies using extensor digitorum longus[78] or tibialis anterior tendon[79] as a free graft, and bone-tendon-bone[80] to reconstruct a chronic deltoid ligament injury have been reported.

It should be noted that many of these reconstruction techniques have been described in relation to the treatment of valgus talar tilt within the ankle mortise for Stage IV TPT insufficiency, which is not compatible with elite sport.[81]

Additional procedures At the time of deltoid ligament surgery, the integrity of the TPT and spring ligament should be assessed. Degenerate lesions can be debrided, tears and splits repaired, lengthened tendons and ligaments shortened, and dysfunctional tendons reinforced with an FDL transfer.

In chronic medial instability, reconstructed soft tissue can be protected with the addition of a calcaneal osteotomy. Either a medial displacement osteotomy to improve a valgus hindfoot or a lateral column lengthening to correct a combined hindfoot valgus/abduction forefoot deformity can be performed. While improving foot mechanics, the addition of an osteotomy adds to potential morbidity from the procedure and may effect a return to elite sport.

Medial Ligament Impingement

Anterior, posterior, and lateral impingement syndromes of the ankle are well described. Medial ankle soft-tissue impingement is less common. It is secondary to deltoid ligament abnormality and can be either anteromedial or posteromedial. Such impingement can involve elements of the deep[82] and superficial[83] components.

Repeated eversion injuries cause ligament damage in the form of partial tearing, leading to enthesiopathic changes, calcification, and granulation tissue. A thickened, hypervascular structure is created, which causes medial ankle pain and associated stiffness. Similarly inversion injuries can cause damage by compression to the deltoid ligament, creating chronic symptoms. Mosier-La Clair and Monroe[83] considered another etiologic factor to be posttraumatic laxity of the anterior tibiotalar ligament, allowing increased anteroposterior ankle laxity and increased contact pressure of the anteromedial talus against the ligament.

Anteromedial impingement

Anteromedial impingement is due to either the development of a meniscoid lesion, found in front of the anterior tibiotalar ligament, or simple thickening of the ligament itself. The meniscoid lesion can appear as an isolated structure or as attached to damaged fibers from a partially torn ligament. In ankle dorsiflexion, it causes localized pain as the lesion impinges on the talus. It may lead to the development of osteophytes in the anteromedial corner of the joint or osteochondral lesion of the talus.[84–86] Jowett and colleagues[87] described 5 elite athletes presenting in 3 years with a medial malleolar stress fracture in association with an anteromedial tibial spur and history of chronic anteromedial impingement.

Posteromedial impingement

Posteromedial impingement follows a significant inversion injury. The deep posterior tibiotalar fibers are compressed and crushed between the medial talar wall and the posterior margin of the medial malleolus, causing contusion, inflammation, and scarring. The initial, often predominant, lateral ligament symptoms settle and the patient is aware of remaining, localized posteromedial pain from the thickened, impinging fibers of deep ligament.[88]

MRI, especially arthrography, can demonstrate thickening of the damaged fibers and any bone edema, caused by friction on the neighboring osteochondral structures, meniscoid lesions, and other associated lesions.

Diagnostic injections of local anesthetic (most accurately placed under ultrasound guidance) can be helpful in confirming the diagnosis.

Surgery for medial impingement

For intractable cases that fail to resolve, the patient's ankle should be examined for stability and arthroscopy undertaken to identify and excise any identified lesion. Mosier-La Clair and Monroe[83] described a small anteromedial arthrotomy to partially excise the thickened ligament, excise osteophytes and synovial tissue, and tidy up chondral lesions. Paterson and colleagues[88] described a combination of ankle arthroscopy, usually combined with a posteromedial arthrotomy through the TPT bed, to visualize the abnormality and allow adequate excision.

Osseous Abnormalities at the Medial Malleolar Tip

Plain radiographs of athletes will frequently show abnormalities at the tip of the medial malleolus. Coral[89] found accessory bones in the subtibial area in 4.6% of 700 ankle radiographs.

Early degenerative changes within the ankle mortise are often associated with a change from a rounded to sharpened tip of the medial malleolus. Previous medial malleolar fractures can be associated with altered geometry and new bone formation (**Fig. 7**).

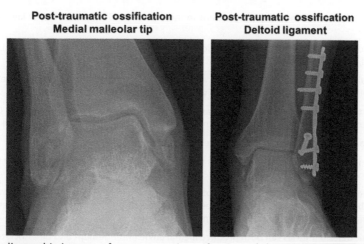

Post-traumatic ossification
Medial malleolar tip

Post-traumatic ossification
Deltoid ligament

Fig. 7. Radiographic images of posttraumatic ossification of the medial malleolar tip and deltoid ligament.

For accessory ossicles and/or ossification, the differential diagnosis should include:

- Avulsion fractures of the medial malleolus
- Unrecognized medial malleolar stress fracture[87]
- Posttraumatic ossification of the deltoid ligament complex (see **Fig. 7**)
- Partial or complete avulsion of the deltoid ligament complex
- Os subtibiale
- Accessory ossification center
- Periosteal response to posteromedial impingement[88]

Deltoid ligament injuries can induce ossification within the thickened fibers. Similar to the lateral malleolus, avulsion fractures can occur medially and remain not united. These avulsion fractures generally arise from the anterior colliculus of the malleolus. Anterior ossicles are present in 2.1% of the population.[89]

The os subtibiale is an accessory ossicle found immediately distal to the medial malleolar tip. It varies in shape and size, and can be confused with any of the afore-mentioned. In comparison with avulsion fractures, this ossicle is located next to posterior colliculus. It is usually greater than 4 mm in diameter and well rounded,[89] being found in up to 1.2% of the population.[90]

Rarely an unfused malleolar accessory ossification center, which are generally smaller than an os subtibiale and found anteriorly, may be seen. These lesions are usually rounded in comparison with avulsion injuries or deltoid ossification, which are usually more irregular. Usually the ossification center is fully fused to the medial malleolus by the age of 11 years. Powell[91] found such ossicles in 2 of 50 adults (4%), with no evidence of ankle trauma.

When such appearances are seen on plain radiographs in association with medial ankle pain, it can be difficult to assess their contribution to the clinical picture. CT scans can be helpful in determining a likely cause and accurate location. Single-photon emission CT (SPECT) can increase predictability as to their likely contribution to the patient's pain.

In the young athlete it is important to distinguish between an avulsion fracture, ligament avulsion, unfused ossification centers, and an os subtibiale. Even in the

---

Learning points for deltoid ligament injuries in elite sport

- Isolated deltoid ligament injuries account for no more than 3% to 4% of all ankle ligament injuries.

- More commonly they occur in conjunction with fractures or other ligament injuries: spring, lateral, and syndesmotic.

- Clinical features include medial pain and tenderness in conjunction with a feeling of instability. The foot assumes a progressive valgus hindfoot and pronated position.

- Stress testing in combination injuries can help document the degree of instability. Chronic cases often show valgus tilt within the ankle mortise for which stress testing has little to add.

- MRI can help define the extent and level of the injury.

- Acute isolated deltoid ligament injuries that are promptly diagnosed can usually be treated conservatively.

- For chronic deltoid instability, a variety of methods of repair and/or reconstruction have been described, although most reported series are in conjunction with more severe grades of TPT dysfunction rather than in high-performance athletes.

- Chronic deltoid injuries can both produce medial ankle impingement and be associated with various osseous abnormalities at the medial malleolar tip.

presence of a fracture, a period of rest and immobilization to settle symptoms should be initiated before consideration is given to surgical excision.

TIBIALIS POSTERIOR TENDON
Anatomy

The tibialis posterior (TP) muscle is a bipenniform muscle, which arises from the posterior surfaces of the tibia (distal to the soleal line) and the fibula, and the intervening interosseous membrane. Despite its short excursion of approximately 2 cm, the TP is a strong muscle, estimated as variably possessing 13% to 23% of triceps surae strength.[92,93]

The tendon (TPT) commences in the lower quarter of the deep posterior compartment of the leg. It runs within a fibrous tunnel and is enveloped in a synovial sheath that commences 6 cm proximal to the medial malleolus and continues for 7 to 9 cm to the navicular tuberosity. During anatomic dissections, Van Dijk and colleagues[94] described the presence of vinculae attached to the TPT similar to those described in the flexor tendon sheaths of the fingers. These mesotendinous structures extend from the tendon to the tendon sheath and adjoining sheath of the FDL. The investigators postulated that the vinculae may become thickened after trauma, interfering with tendon function and creating pain. Their presence was confirmed during endoscopy, and the release of particularly thickened vinculae was reported as providing relief of symptoms in correctly identified patients.

Proximally and distally the tendon receives a satisfactory vascular supply from the muscular branches of the posterior tibial artery and the periosteal vessels, respectively, of the navicular communicating with the longitudinal tendon vessels. In between is a length of approximately 14 to 15 mm, starting 15 mm distal to the medial malleolus and extending proximally, where the tendon's synovial sheath is relatively hypovascular. It is this short segment that has been associated with the site of pathologic change including attritional rupture.[95]

The insertion of TPT is extensive. Bloome and colleagues[96] described 3 insertional bands (**Table 3**).

Function and Biomechanics

The TPT inverts the hindfoot and adducts the forefoot by balancing the activity of the peroneus brevis. At heel strike during gait, the TPT eccentrically contracts to control hindfoot eversion, working as a shock absorber across the subtalar joint.[97] By midstance, the TPT has inverted the heel and locked the transverse tarsal joint as a stable

Table 3
Tibialis posterior tendon insertions

Name	Tendon Width (%)	Insertions
Anterior	65	Navicular tuberosity Inferior naviculocuneiform joint capsule Inferior middle cuneiform
Middle	15	Middle and lateral cuneiforms Cuboid Metatarsals II–IV
Posterior	20	Contributes to the acetabulum pedis

Data from Bloome DM, Marymont JV, Varner KE. Variations on the insertion of the posterior tibialis tendon: a cadaveric study. Foot Ankle Int 2003;24(10):780–3.

construct to produce a rigid lever for the gastrocnemius-soleus complex, thus to propel the foot forward, acting at the level of the metatarsal heads.

As the foot is propelled forward, the TPT further supinates the subtalar joint and helps initiate heel lift. Having worked synergistically with the peroneal muscles to allow the translation of the center of body weight from lateral to medial, the PTT reduces activity following heel lift.

Tendon dysfunction causes profound changes in foot biomechanics. With hindfoot inversion reduced and a failure to lock the transverse tarsal joint during midstance, a more unstable construct is produced, preventing the development of a rigid lever. Consequently the point of action of the gastrocnemius-soleus complex is transferred proximally from the metatarsal heads to act on the talonavicular joint. The midfoot becomes increasingly abducted, and increased strain is placed at Lisfranc level. Propulsive strength is reduced with delayed heel lift and less loading of the lateral structures. The increasing load on the supporting structures, including the spring ligament, will eventually cause degeneration and failure. Once the spring ligament fails to cradle the talar head, the latter will plantarflex and the heel adopt an increasingly valgus alignment. The navicular is allowed to rotate laterally around the talus, producing forefoot abduction.

Tibialis Posterior Dysfunction

Abnormalities of the TPT complex in the athlete can involve several potential pathologic factors. Advanced grades of TP insufficiency with their concomitant deformities are not compatible with elite performance. The management of these latter stages are more likely to be seen in the older patient, dealt with extensively in the literature and, therefore, not covered in this article.

Since Johnson and Strom[98] first classified 3 stages of TP dysfunction in 1989, various investigators have refined it further, and Myerson's[99] 4-stage classification containing various substages is recognized as a useful means of evaluation and guide for management.

Stage I disease

In Stage I disease, the athlete complains of discomfort and swelling along the path of the TPT. Often no single initiating episode is recognized. Symptoms frequently will extend more proximally within the muscle on the posteromedial aspect of the calf. Symptoms will routinely be aggravated by training. Observation of the limb will often reveal a planus foot position, but with no or minimal hindfoot valgus ($\leq 5°$) or forefoot abduction. Tenderness and swelling can be elicited anywhere from the navicular tuberosity to the musculotendinous junction and beyond. The patient can tiptoe in both double stance and single stance, bringing the hindfoot into varus during the process. Some patients will have a mild to moderate accompanying hallux valgus deformity. Formal testing of the TP strength on resisted activity with the foot held in plantarflexion and inversion will reveal an intact tendon, although pain may limit full resistance.

For patients (even elite athletes) presenting with significant synovial inflammation within the TPT sheath, the possibility of other diagnoses, such as rheumatoid arthritis and seronegative inflammatory conditions (eg, gout), should be entertained. The appropriate investigations should be undertaken as part of the initial workup. Inflammatory causation was recognized by Myerson[99] as a separate entity (Stage IA). A neutral hindfoot warrants a staging of IB and with mild hindfoot valgus positioning, Stage IC.

Tenosynovitis was barely recognized in this tendon until the 1970s. In the absence of some form of systemic inflammatory disease, Myerson and colleagues[100] found it more commonly in the older age group (average age 55 years). Supple and colleagues[101] described the condition in younger athletes, especially those involved in running sports, and associated it with overtraining and rapid repetitive movements, especially those involving direction changes. Overloading of the medial structures including the TPT, deltoid ligament, and spring ligament complex during impact activity, especially sport, can induce inflammation within the tendon sheath and micro-tears to the tendon at activity levels of 1500 to 2000 cycles per hour.[102] Synovial thickening and increased fluid production follow.

At this stage, the paratenon is inflamed and the tendon may be thickened with small splits or longitudinal tears while retaining its overall integrity and length. With chronicity, the sheath may thicken and adhesions form, affecting tendon excursion and efficiency.[103] The tendon within the sheath may feel stenosed and the vinculae[94] thickened.

The infiltration of local anesthetic into the sheath for diagnosis when doubt exists as to the cause of pain (even after imaging), with or without ultrasound guidance, has been reported as an accurate, safe, and sensitive modality.[104]

Imaging In Stage I disease the overall alignment of the foot and ankle should appear normal on radiography, but other modalities are required to rule out other anomalies such as an accessory navicular or some form of tarsal coalition.

Tenography may help in identifying sheath tenosynovitis or stenosis. However, its ability to accurately diagnose tendon abnormality correlates poorly with surgical findings[105] and has been superseded by other imaging modalities.

Ultrasonography is useful in distinguishing between the various stages of TP dysfunction. In tenosynovitis, ultrasonography will demonstrate the degree of fluid surrounding the tendon and thickening of the tendon (normal diameter 4–6 mm).[106] It will demonstrate any irregular form seen in tendinosis or longitudinal splits. The fluid will widen the synovial sheath. As the disease progresses to Stages II and III, the amount of sheath fluid often diminishes as tendon size increases, and splits, tears, and tendon lengthening are more likely to be seen (**Fig. 8**).[107] Hypervascularity associated with acute inflammatory changes will be demonstrated using the Doppler signal on ultrasonography.

Like ultrasonography, MRI is excellent at demonstrating normal and abnormal anatomy of the TPT and sheath for the features outlined here. In addition, MRI is superior in demonstrating abnormalities of the spring and deltoid ligament complex. It can demonstrate bone edema and early articular damage, and its sensitivity allows it

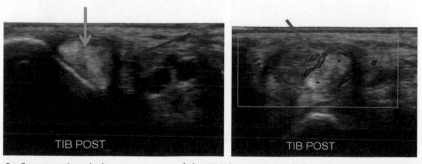

Fig. 8. Cross-sectional ultrasonograms of the TPT (*green arrow*) showing tenosynovitis (*blue arrow*) and hypervascularity on Doppler signal (*red arrow*).

to identify intrasubstance tears that may not be appreciated during perioperative inspection (**Fig. 9**).[99]

Treatment

Conservative Treatment of Stage I disease will initially be conservative. A review with the athlete and coaching staff will be helpful in identifying any underlying technical problems that may have initiated or exacerbated the problem.

Alvarez and colleagues[108] highlighted the paucity of publications on the conservative management of Stage I and Stage II TPT dysfunction, with only 4 previous reports.

Simple measures such as initial cessation from repetitive loading activities, cryotherapy, and nonsteroidal anti-inflammatories (NSAIDs) either topically (iontophoresis) or orally will help control the release of noxious mediators of inflammation.[109]

Early immobilization in a removable walking boot is helpful and can be supplemented with an orthotic to support the arch. In addition, it allows access for physiotherapy. Once the acute symptoms have settled, the boot is removed but the foot benefits from continuing support whether with an in-shoe orthotic or something more substantial such as an Airlift PTTD Brace (DJO, Carlsbad, CA). Functional deficits should be sought. Alvarez and colleagues[108] noted a common feature of weakness and imbalance combined with a tight gastrocnemius-soleus complex. In the athlete any identified weakness may be relative, but clearly below the level required for the particular sporting activity. Alvarez and colleagues[108] laid down strict criteria for completion of rehabilitation, but these pertained to nonelite athletes, and return to activity is dependent on the particular demands of each sport.

Steroids The use of oral steroids, in the absence of systemic disease, and sheath injections for tenosynovitis carries a significant risk of complications, particularly rupture. Holmes and Mann[110] reported that local infiltration may adversely affect vascular supply within the sheath and that 28% of younger patients presenting with TP rupture had received either oral corticosteroids or repeated injections. Johnson and Strom[98] expressed similar safety concerns. In addition, athletes, by the nature of their sports, often have low body mass indices with minimal subcutaneous fat. Local steroid injections around the foot and ankle may produce unsightly subcutaneous fat atrophy and hypopigmentation.

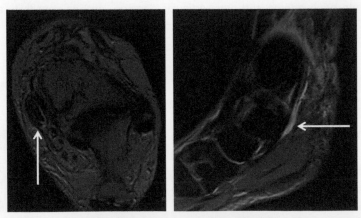

Fig. 9. MRI axial and sagittal sections demonstrating TPT split and tenosynovitis (*white arrows*).

High-volume stripping In cases where there is considered to be a degree of scarring, stenosis, or thickened vinculae with no obvious tendon tears or splits, the senior author (W.R.) has found that ultrasound-guided infiltration of the sheath with saline to free the tendon followed by physiotherapy has been useful in relieving pain and dysfunction.

Surgery Failure of conservative treatment warrants consideration of the surgical options. Myerson's[100] suggestion of surgical intervention after 3 months of nonresponse to conservative measures seems reasonable.

The timing of such intervention varies according to perceived pathology and etiology. For athletes with mechanical overload, more time should be allowed to assess the outcome of conservative treatment than for patients with systemic inflammatory disease. However, if imaging reveals the possibility of early longitudinal tears, earlier intervention should be considered.

Tenosynovectomy If conservative treatment fails and no structural deformity is present, surgical decompression and tenosynovectomy can be performed. Surgical intervention can be open or endoscopic.

Tibialis posterior tendinoscopy The use of hindfoot endoscopy for diagnostic and therapeutic procedures was established by van Dijk and colleagues.[94] The TPT can be accessed endoscopically by a 2-portal technique. Van Dijk and colleagues have described its use in the resection of thickened vinculae, synovectomy, tendon sheath release, postfracture metalwork removal, and loose-body extraction. Other workers have described its use in diagnosis and the treatment of tendon conditions including synovectomy, adhesion release, stenosis, and the treatment of partial lesions.[111] Chow and colleagues,[112] in a small series, reported the outcome for tenosynovectomy as equal to that for open procedure.

Open synovectomy Formal exposure of the tendon should take place from the navicular tuberosity proximal to the medial malleolus. Once the sheath is open, its contents should be carefully inspected. A thorough synovectomy is undertaken and specimens sent for histology. Sheath closure should be undertaken meticulously with respect to obtaining correct tension to stop tendon dislocation while preventing tendon stenosis.

Splits should be debrided and repaired. Significant longitudinal tears should be repaired and the TPT supplemented with an FDL transfer (**Fig. 10**).[113]

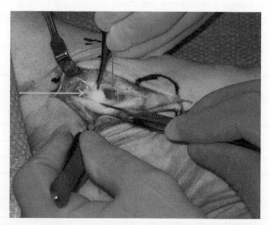

Fig. 10. Arrows indicate tibialis posterior tenosynovitis and tendinosis with longitudinal splits.

Stage II disease

By the time the athlete has reached Stage II disease, the TPT has undergone further degeneration and elongation. The hindfoot displays a valgus position which, however, remains supple and passively correctable. The medial arch collapses and forefoot deformity progresses. Marks and Schon[114] described a young basketball player with a distal TPT intrasubstance tear causing elongation and functional incompetency. The athlete required tendon advancement and protection with a medializing calcaneal osteotomy. The disease can progress to complete rupture.

Myerson[99] subdivided Stage II patients further (Table 4). It is unlikely that an athlete would be able to perform at an elite level by the time substage C has been reached.

Imaging Radiographs will be examined for parameters such as the talar–first metatarsal (Meary) angle, calcaneal pitch, talocalcaneal angle, and medial and lateral column heights, on lateral weight-bearing films. On AP weight-bearing films, the talar–first metatarsal angle and talonavicular uncoverage angle are assessed.

As in Stage I disease, ultrasonography and MRI have their place in assessing soft tissues, including the spring and deltoid ligaments as well as the TPT itself.

Treatment Although conservative treatment may be tried initially, return to the higher echelons of sport is unlikely to be regained without surgical intervention.

Surgery Simple synovectomy and repair of the TPT is inadequate once the tendon has pathologically elongated. Secondary structures such as the spring ligament will come under increased strain.

The diseased TPT needs to be augmented with an FDL transfer and protected with the addition of a calcaneal osteotomy. In athletes at substage A1, a medial calcaneal displacement osteotomy (MCDO) is undertaken. Persistence of a forefoot varus, unless the ankle is plantarflexed, indicates a tight calf complex. Postoperative physiotherapy might address this issue; alternatively surgical correction is performed, a gastrocnemius recession being preferred to percutaneous Achilles tendon lengthening for an elite athlete.

A substage A2 presentation displays a fixed forefoot varus deformity regardless of ankle position. Such a rigid deformity needs correction using a medial cuneiform opening wedge Cotton osteotomy.

By the time further Stage II levels are reached, significant further surgery is required in terms of lateral column lengthening (substage B) and consideration for stabilizing medial column fusion (substage C).

Other abnormalities such as spring ligament attritional rupture should be addressed.

Table 4		
Myerson's tibialis posterior tendon dysfunction Stage II substages (1997)		
Substage	Hindfoot	Forefoot
A1		Flexible varus
A2	Supple valgus	Fixed varus
B		Abduction
C		Fixed varus
		Medial column instability
		First-ray dorsiflexion on hindfoot correction

Data from Bloome DM, Marymont JV, Varner KE. Variations on the insertion of the posterior tibialis tendon: a cadaveric study. Foot Ankle Int 2003;24(10):780–3.

The use of a subtalar arthroereisis implant to supplement surgery has been used successfully in adults and children. This implant blocks excessive subtalar eversion, supports the talar neck, and protects the medial soft-tissue repair(s). Later implant removal for sinus tarsi pain is required in a high percentage of patients (42%), but without loss of corrected position if it has been in place for at least 8 months.[115] The implant can be used instead of an MCDO in milder cases and in conjunction with an MCDO in more advanced cases. VanAman and Schon[116] described the indications for each. Athletes should be made aware of the potential for sinus tarsi pain and the later requirement for implant removal.

No major series exists reporting on return to elite sport after surgical treatment for Stage II disease. Athletes need to be counseled that such extensive surgery is primarily directed at correcting deformity and safeguarding the foot in future. Rehabilitation is prolonged over a period of at least 12 months, and return to high-impact elite sport is unlikely and probably not advised.

Tibialis Posterior Laceration and Acute Rupture

Acute injuries to the TPT during sport are relatively uncommon.

Lacerations to the TPT are rare.[117] In the senior author's (W.R.) experience, lacerations have been witnessed in ice-related sports (eg, speed skating) whereby the skate blades can cause injuries around the ankle. Partial or complete lacerations to the TPT can occur in isolation or in association with injuries to the neighboring tendons and neurovascular structures. The tendon is usually healthy before injury, and can be primarily sutured following suitable wound debridement. Undiagnosed and untreated lacerations can lead to pes planus, even in young patients,[118] requiring reconstruction.

Acute ruptures can occur in combination with ankle fractures, particularly after pronation–external rotation injuries.[119–123] If the exposure is limited medially to expose the fracture only, the tendon injury may be missed. The tendon is usually macroscopically normal apart from the acute injury. Direct tendon repair followed by suitable protection will prevent the development of later planovalgus deformity.

Isolated acute ruptures of the TPT in athletes are rare.[103,124–127] Whereas the middle-aged runner not infrequently presents with TPT problems,[126] presentations in the age group younger than 30 years, especially of acute rupture, are rare.[113] Even in the younger athlete, a history of a previous more minor problem can often be elicited and, at exploration, may show evidence of chronic degeneration that preceded rupture.[113] Surgical treatment should follow the guidelines outlined in the section on Stage II TPT dysfunction.

Tibialis Posterior Dislocation

Compared with peroneal tendon dislocations on the lateral side of the ankle, medial dislocation of the TPT is an unusual injury. It was first described in 1874,[128] with the first description in an English-language journal in 1968.[129]

In association with ankle fractures

The tendon may dislocate in association with ankle fractures and act as a block to reduction.[122,130–132] Suspicion should be aroused if normal ankle anatomy cannot be restored by manipulation and internal fixation of the fracture elements. The tendon will have to be exposed, inspected for any injury, reduced, and stabilized into its anatomic position within its sheath.

Isolated injuries

Isolated tendon dislocations are much less common. Rarely the patient may present with tendon dislocation spontaneously,[133] but the overwhelming majority occur following injury. The mechanism of injury is usually a forced ankle dorsiflexion injury in association with hindfoot inversion leading to failure of the restraining flexor retinaculum. Such an injury in association with an Achilles tendon rupture has been reported.[134] A case of iatrogenic causation has been published following tarsal tunnel release.[135]

A comprehensive literature review reported that 58.5% of such injuries occurred during sport.[136] Several sporting activities have been associated with this injury, including rock-climbing,[136,137] Tae-Kwon-Do,[138] motorcycling,[129] and dance.[139]

Like peroneal tendon instability, some publications have remarked on the variation in sulcus anatomy on the posterior aspect of the medial malleolus as a contributor to potential dislocation. A cadaveric study demonstrated a range of sulcus width from 6 to 15 mm and depth of 1.5 to 4 mm.[140]

It has been reported that 53.1% of patients were misdiagnosed initially,[136] but in the elite athlete, with rapid access to experienced clinicians and imaging, the diagnosis should be made soon after injury.

The athlete will usually be able to confirm the mechanism of injury. In the acute situation, tenderness, swelling, and bruising will often be present posterior and inferior to the medial malleolus. Once the acute symptoms have settled, the patient may complain of instability, localized swelling and discomfort, and intermittent snapping or popping.

Imaging with either ultrasonography or MRI will be able to confirm the diagnosis. Rents in the tendon sheath and fluid around the tendon can be seen. The tendon can be assessed for evidence of tendinopathy, splits, and tears.[136] Deltoid ligament injury[137] and lateral talar dome injury[136] can occur at the same time.

Conservative treatment of this condition by rest and immobilization may be possible if the diagnosis is made promptly in the acute situation. However, Loncarich and Clapper[137] suggest that nonsurgical treatment is uniformly unsuccessful, and the review of the literature by Lohrer and Nauck[136] reported that 83% of patients required operative stabilization.

A range of operative procedures has been described. The review by Lohrer and Nauck[136] summarized the options, which are reproduced in **Table 5**.

Table 5
Surgical options for tibialis posterior dislocation

Technique	Details	% of Cases (N = 49)
Retinaculum repair	Direct suturing	32.7
Retinaculum reefing	To periosteum To suture anchors Intraosseous reefing	18.4

Retinaculum reinforcement/
supplementation
	Inverted periosteal flap retinaculum
	  reconstruction
	Achilles tendon flap retinaculum
	  reconstruction
	Deltoid ligament flap retinaculum
	  reconstruction
	Sliding medial malleolus reconstruction
		24.5

Groove deepening	Combined with retinaculum repair or reconstruction	18.4
Posterior tibial tendon decompression only	No attempt to correct instability	2.0
Not specified		4.1

Data from Lohrer H, Nauck T. Posterior tibial tendon dislocation: a systematic review of the literature and presentation of a case. Br J Sports Med 2010;44(6)398–406.

The literature review[136] revealed that surgical outcomes were reported as excellent in 80% and good in a further 12%. However, as the largest 2 case series reported comprised only 7 patients,[141,142] the optimal surgical option remains to be determined, with no individual surgeon gaining sufficient experience to be able to publish a major series.

Accessory Navicular

A common cause of pain in the athlete is related to the presence of the accessory navicular, or os tibiale externum. It is the most common ossicle in the foot,[143] and its reported incidence varies from between 2% and 14% of the population.[144–146]

Such injuries have been classified by various investigators since Dwight's[147] first description in 1907 **(Table 6)**.[148–151]

Type 1 abnormalities are rarely of clinical importance. Most clinical problems arise from Type 2 accessory navicular.

Imaging

Plain radiographs consisting of AP and lateral weight-bearing views with an additional 45° external oblique view will confirm the clinical impression of an accessory navicular, and allow typing. Radiography allows review of overall foot alignment, particularly with respect to planovalgus deformities. In cases of clinical doubt, plain radiographs can be supplemented by other modalities, for instance when distinguishing between a Type 2 accessory ossicle and suspected tuberosity fractures, and when further information is required concerning the distal part of the TPT.

Isotope scanning will demonstrate increased uptake at the synchondrosis, but nowadays this is more commonly replaced by other imaging modalities.

MRI will demonstrate bone edema on either side of the synchondrosis in symptomatic ossicles, often with enhancement and thickening at the tendon insertion. Wong and Griffith[152] described it as an enthesiopathy type appearance.

Ultrasonography will define PTT damage, can demonstrate increased vascularity around the symptomatic area, and may be useful for guiding diagnostic or therapeutic injections.[153]

CT will define the osseous anatomy well and will help to differentiate fractures from ossicles. SPECT allows confirmation of the site of pain.[154]

Table 6
Classification of accessory navicular types

Type	Subtype	Description	Comments
1		Sesamoid in the posterior tibial tendon	30% of cases
			Round or oval-shaped and distinct from tuberosity. Plantar position close to the inferior part of the spring ligament
2		Articulating accessory ossification center	Separated from main body by fibrocartilaginous plate (synchondrosis)
			Often irregular
	2a		Connected to body at a less acute angle than 2b. Ossicle is subjected primarily to a tension forces
	2b		Situated more inferiorly than 2a and more subjected to shearing forces
3		Fused accessory ossification center	A ridge is often found at point of fusion

Treatment

Some patients present for advice regarding the significance of the excessive, albeit asymptomatic, bony prominence, requiring no more than reassurance. Others will present because of pain.

A clear traumatic episode can be rested in a below-knee weight-bearing cast until the worst of symptoms have settled. Later, molded orthotics providing heel and medial arch support can be provided.

Symptoms arising more insidiously require careful appraisal and explanation to the athlete. Rest and cessation of those aspects of their sport that aggravate the problem should be advised. Review of normal and sports footwear may reveal shoe uppers that cause rubbing and friction. Shoes with greater width and appropriate support should be advised. Pain is usually caused by forces, whether they be tension, shear, or compression, transmitted through the insertion of the tendon to the synchondrosis. Initial rest in a removable walker can help initially.

NSAIDs can provide short-term relief. Rarely, ultrasound-guided steroid injections placed accurately at the synchondrosis followed by a period of rest are required in resistant cases. Patients should be advised of the possibility of tendon weakening following injection.

Once again during the recovery period, biomechanical assessment and orthotic provision should be organized to diminish the risk of recurrence.

In those athletes failing a reasonable period of conservative treatment, surgery has to be considered. The range of surgical options and outcomes has been well summarized by Leonard and Fortin,[155] and are outlined in **Table 7**.

Small painful Type 2 ossicles respond well to simple excision. A variety of approaches to the ossicle through the TPT has been described.[145,156–158] Whichever

Table 7		
Surgical options for symptomatic accessory navicular		
Excision	± Plication of the mobilized tendon	For small ossicles and no significant planovalgus deformity
	PLUS rerouting the tibialis posterior tendon into a more plantar position	Original Kidner procedure.[153,154]
	PLUS suturing of the tendon into the freshened bed of the navicular	
	PLUS tendon continuity restoration	
Percutaneous drilling across synchondrosis		To attempt to induce union across the synchondrosis
Arthrodesis of the ossicle to the main navicular body		For larger ossicles
Accessory procedures to realign planovalgus foot	Correction of gastrocsoleus tightness	
	Medial displacement calcaneal osteotomy	
	Lateral column lengthening	
	Subtalar arthroereisis	

Data from Wong MW, Griffith JF. Magnetic imaging in adolescent painful flexible flatfoot. Foot Ankle Int 2009;30(4):303–8.

approach is used, it is important to inspect the integrity of the tendon and ensure it is properly reconstructed at the end of the procedure.

Kidner[159,160] advocated rerouting the TPT into a more inferior position after excising the accessory navicular to restore the "normal line of pull." Although subsequent published results have demonstrated good outcomes, there is some doubt as to whether the procedure improves arch position and whether there is any advantage over simple excision and in situ repair of the tendon.[149,161]

Young athletes were treated by the simple, minimally invasive procedure of percutaneous drilling by Nakayama and colleagues,[162] with only 1 failure in 31 patients. Pain relief is believed to be achieved by inducing bone union across the synchondrosis. However, further series have yet to be published.

Larger accessory navicular can be considered for taking down of the synchondrosis, reducing any excessive prominence from the main body of the navicular, advancing the PTT distally and inferiorly, and achieving union by stabilizing with screw fixation. Although some nonunions have been reported, overall patient satisfaction and return to sport are claimed to be as high as for other techniques.[163–165]

Learning points for TPT injuries in elite sport

- TPT dysfunction presenting in the elite athlete usually occurs at the Stage I level.

- However, other problems may arise in relation to its insertion, particularly with an accessory navicular and, more rarely, catastrophic failure causing tendon dislocation and even rupture.

- Careful clinical evaluation supported by appropriate imaging should be undertaken to clarify the nature of the damage and, for TPT dysfunction, stage the disability.

- Most insertional and early tendon abnormalities can be treated conservatively, with attention to underlying biomechanical and technical deficits.

- Surgical interventions should only be considered after an adequate period of assessment and conservative treatment. In the absence of significant disability, simple synovectomy and decompression may suffice.

- However, for more advanced tendon disease, insertional abnormality, and instability or rupture, surgical intervention becomes more involved with careful counseling regarding the recovery program and return to elite sport.

- For spring and deltoid abnormality, there is a dearth of major published literature on outcomes of both conservative and surgical procedures in elite athletes.

SUMMARY

Injuries to the medial side of the ankle and hindfoot involving one or more of the spring ligament, deltoid ligament, and TPT can occur in isolation or in combination with other bone and ligament damage. Individual injuries to the spring and deltoid ligaments are comparatively rare, whereas TPT dysfunction is relatively common.

Elite athletes will usually present with early Stage I and II TPT disease. Prompt diagnosis and management is intended to not only return athletes to their previous level of sport but also prevent deterioration to levels incompatible with return to play. During the rehabilitation phase, an analysis of the individual athlete to identify biomechanical and technical deficits contributing to the initial problem is helpful in allowing prophylactic measures to be introduced. In addition, unrecognized or untreated TPT disease can cause secondary injury to the complexes of both the spring and deltoid ligaments.

Isolated deltoid injuries promptly diagnosed can usually be treated conservatively, but chronic injury and combination abnormality often require surgical intervention. Complete spring ligament injuries, particularly to the SMCNL segment, require operative intervention and, usually, reinforcement in combination with the treatment of any concomitant abnormality.

However, published data on both the conservative and surgical management of damage to these 3 medial structures is sparse. Treatment decisions require extrapolating data from patient series predominantly including nonathletes and recreational athletes and placing such information in the context of the demands of each sport, with appropriate rehabilitation schedules designed accordingly.

REFERENCES

1. Bluman EM, Title CI, Myerson MS. Posterior tibial tendon rupture: a refined classification system. Foot Ankle Clin 2007;12(2):233–49.
2. Sarrafian SK. Anatomy of the foot and ankle: descriptive, topographic, functional. Philadelphia: Lippincott; 1983. p. 159–282.
3. Patil V, Ebraheim NA, Frogameni A, et al. Morphometric dimensions of the calcaneonavicular (spring) ligament. Foot Ankle Int 2007;28(8):927–32.
4. Taniguchi A, Tanaka Y, Takakura Y, et al. Anatomy of the spring ligament. J Bone Joint Surg Am 2003;85:2174–8.
5. Kitaoka HB, Ahn TK, Luo ZP, et al. Stability of the arch of the foot. Foot Ankle Int 1997;18:644–8.
6. Iaquinto JM, Wayne JS. Computational model of the lower leg and foot/ankle complex: application to arch stability. J Biomech Eng 2010;132(2): 021009.
7. Hollinshead WH. Anatomy for surgeons, vol. 3. New York: Hoeber-Harper; 1954. p. 831–81.
8. Davis WH, Sobel M, DiCarlo EF, et al. Gross, histological, and microvascular anatomy and biomechanical testing of the spring ligament complex. Foot Ankle Int 1996;17:95–102.
9. Jennings MM, Christensen JC. The effects of sectioning the spring ligament on rearfoot stability and posterior tibial tendon efficiency. J Foot Ankle Surg 2008; 47(3):219–24.
10. Deland JT. The adult acquired flatfoot and spring ligament complex. Foot Ankle Clin 2001;6(1):129–35.
11. Gazdag AR, Cracchiolo A. Rupture of the posterior tibial tendon. Evaluation of injury of the spring ligament and clinical assessment of tendon transfer and ligament repair. J Bone Joint Surg Am 1997;79(5):675–81.
12. Balen PE, Helms CA. Association of posterior tibial tendon injury with spring ligament injury, sinus tarsi abnormality and plantar fasciitis on MR imaging. AJR Am J Roentgenol 2001;176(5):1137–43.
13. Borton DC, Saxby TS. Tear of the plantar calcaneonavicular (spring) ligament causing flatfoot. A case report. J Bone Joint Surg Br 1997;79(4):641–3.
14. Chen JP, Allen AM. MR diagnosis of traumatic tear of the spring ligament in a pole vaulter. Skeletal Radiol 1997;26(5):310–2.
15. Subhas N, Sundaram M. Diagnosis: isolated spring ligament tear demonstrated on magnetic resonance imaging. Orthopedics 2007;30(1):70–2.
16. Tryfonidis M, Jackson W, Mansour R, et al. Acquired adult flat foot due to isolated plantar calcaneonavicular (spring) ligament insufficiency with a normal tibialis posterior tendon. Foot Ankle Surg 2008;14(2):89–95.

17. Shuen V, Prem H. Acquired unilateral pes planus in a child caused by a ruptured plantar calcaneonavicular (spring) ligament. J Pediatr Orthop B 2009;18(3):129–30.
18. Kavanagh EC, Koulouris G, Gopez A, et al. MRI of rupture of the spring ligament complex with talo-cuboid impaction. Skeletal Radiol 2007;36(6):555–8.
19. Yao L, Gentili A, Cracchiolo A. MR imaging findings in spring ligament insufficiency. Skeletal Radiol 1999;28(5):245–50.
20. Toye LR, Helms CA, Hoffmann BD, et al. MRI of spring ligament tears. AJR Am J Roentgenol 2005;184(5):1475–80.
21. Hintermann B. Medial ankle instability. Foot Ankle Clin 2003;8(4):723–38.
22. Hintermann B. Treatment of deltoid ligament injuries. In: Hintermann B, editor. Proceedings of Sports Foot and Ankle 2011. Liestal Switzerland: Warwick University; 2011. p. 359–73.
23. Cobey JC. Posterior roentgenogram of the foot. Clin Orthop 1976;118:202–7.
24. Rule J, Yao L, Seeger L. Spring ligament of the ankle: normal MR anatomy. AJR Am J Roentgenol 1993;161:1241–4.
25. Harish S, Jan E, Findlay K, et al. Sonography of the superomedial part of the spring ligament complex of the foot: a study of cadavers and asymptomatic volunteers. Skeletal Radiol 2007;36(3):221–8.
26. Harish S, Kumbhare D, O'Neill J, et al. Comparison of sonography and magnetic resonance imaging for spring ligament abnormalities: preliminary study. J Ultrasound Med 2008;27(8):1145–53.
27. Mann RA. Flatfoot in adults. In: Coughlin MJ, Mann RA, editors. Surgery of the foot and ankle. St Louis (MO): Mosby; 1999. p. 733–67.
28. Hiller L, Pinney SJ. Surgical treatment of acquired adult flatfoot deformity: what is the state of practice among academic foot and ankle surgeons in 2002? Foot Ankle Int 2003;24(9):701–5.
29. Goldner JL, Keats PK, Bassett FH 3rd, et al. Progressive talipes equinovalgus due to trauma or degeneration of the posterior tibial tendon and medial plantar ligaments. Orthop Clin North Am 1974;5:39–51.
30. Deland JT, Annoczky S, Thompson FM. Adult acquired flatfoot deformity at the talonavicular joint: reconstruction of the spring ligament in an in vitro model. Foot Ankle Int 1992;13:327–32.
31. Thordarson DB, Schmotzer H, Chon J. Reconstruction with tenodesis in an adult flatfoot model. A biomechanical evaluation of four methods. J Bone Joint Surg Am 2003;77:1557–64.
32. Choi K, Lee S, Otis JC, et al. Anatomical reconstruction of the spring ligament using peroneus longus tendon graft. Foot Ankle Int 2003;24(5):430–6.
33. Williams BR, Ellis SJ, Deyer TW, et al. Reconstruction of the spring ligament using a peroneus longus autograft tendon transfer. Foot Ankle Int 2010;31(7):567–77.
34. Otis JC, Deland JT, Kenneally SM, et al. Medial arch strain after medial displacement calcaneal osteotomy: an in vitro study. Foot Ankle Int 1999;20(4):222–6.
35. Sarrafian SK. Anatomy of the foot and ankle. 2nd edition. Philadelphia: J.B. Lippincott; 1993. p. 174–85.
36. Milner CE, Soames RW. The medial collateral ligaments of the human ankle joint: anatomical variations. Foot Ankle Int 1998;19:289–92.
37. Boss AP, Hintermann B. Anatomical study of the medial ankle ligament complex. Foot Ankle Int 2002;23:547–53.
38. Close JR. Some applications of the functional anatomy of the ankle joint. J Bone Joint Surg Am 1956;38:761–81.
39. Harper MC. The deltoid ligament: an anatomical evaluation of function. Foot Ankle 1987;8:19–22.

40. Rasmussen O, Kroman-Andersen C, Boe S. Deltoid ligament: functional analysis of the medial collateral ligamentous apparatus of the ankle joint. Acta Orthop Scand 1983;54:36–44.

41. Michelson JD, Ahn UM, Helgemo SL. Motion of the ankle in a simulated supination-external rotation fracture. J Bone Joint Surg Am 1996;78:1024–31.

42. Michelson JD, Waldman B. An axially loaded model of the ankle after pronation external rotation injury. Clin Orthop Relat Res 1996;328:285–93.

43. Attarian DE, McCrakin HJ, DeVito DP, et al. Biomechanical characteristics of human ankle ligaments. Foot Ankle 1985;6(2):54–8.

44. Beumer A, van Hemert WL, Swierstra BA, et al. A biomechanical evaluation of the tibiofibular and tibiotalar ligaments of the ankle. Foot Ankle Int 2003;24(5): 426–9.

45. Bröstrum L. Sprained ankles. I. Anatomic lesions in recent sprains. Acta Chir Scand 1964;128:483–95.

46. Gerber JP, Williams GN, Scoville CR, et al. Persistent disability associated with ankle sprains: a prospective examination of an athletic population. Foot Ankle Int 1998;19:653–60.

47. Jackson R, Willis RE. Rupture of deltoid ligament without involvement of the lateral ligament. Am J Sports Med 1988;16:541–3.

48. McConley JP, Lloyd-Smith R, Li D. Complete rupture of the deltoid ligament of the ankle. Clin J Sport Med 1991;1:133–7.

49. Harper MC. The deltoid ligament. An evaluation of function and need for surgical repair. Clin Orthop Relat Res 1988;226:156–68.

50. Hintermann B, Regazzoni P, Lampert C, et al. Arthroscopic findings in acute fractures of the ankle. J Bone Joint Surg Br 2000;82:345–51.

51. Miller CD, Shelton WR, Barett GR, et al. Deltoid and syndesmosis ligament injury of the ankle without fracture. Am J Sports Med 1995;23:746–50.

52. Tornetta P III. Competence of the deltoid ligament in bimalleolar ankle fractures after medial malleolar fixation. J Bone Joint Surg Am 2000;82:843–8.

53. Gougoulias N, Khanna A, Sakellariou A, et al. Supination-external rotation ankle fractures: stability a key issue. Clin Orthop Relat Res 2010;468(1):243–51.

54. van den Bekerom MP, Mutsaerts EL, van Dijk CN. Evaluation of the integrity of the deltoid ligament in supination external rotation ankle fractures: a systematic review of the literature. Arch Orthop Trauma Surg 2009;129(2):227–35.

55. DeAngelis NA, Eskander MS, French BG. Does medial tenderness predict deep deltoid ligament incompetence in supination-external rotation type ankle fractures? J Orthop Trauma 2007;21(4):244–7.

56. Maynou C, Lesage P, Mestdagh H, et al. Is surgical treatment of deltoid ligament rupture necessary in ankle fractures? Rev Chir Orthop Reparatrice Appar Mot 1997;83(7):652–7.

57. Crim JR, Beals TC, Nickisch F, et al. Deltoid ligament abnormalities in chronic lateral ankle instability. Foot Ankle Int 2011;32(9):873–8.

58. Hintermann B, Boss A, Schafer D. Arthroscopic findings in patients with chronic ankle instability. Am J Sports Med 2002;30(3):402–9.

59. Buchhorn T, Sabeti-Aschraf M, Dlaska CE, et al. Combined medial and lateral anatomic lateral reconstruction for chronic rotational instability of the ankle. Foot Ankle Int 2011;32(12):1122–6.

60. Boytim MJ, Fischer DA, Neumann L. Syndesmotic ankle sprains. Am J Sports Med 1991;19:294–8.

61. Hopkinson WJ, St Pierre P, Ryan JB, et al. Syndesmosis sprains of the ankle. Foot Ankle 1990;10:325–30.

62. Hintermann B, Knupp M, Pagenstert GI. Deltoid ligament injuries: diagnosis and management. Foot Ankle Clin 2006;11(3):625–38.
63. Hintermann B, Valderrrabano V, Boss AP, et al. Medial ankle instability— a prospective study of 54 cases. Am J Sports Med 2004;32(1):183–90.
64. Raikin SM, Myerson MS. Surgical repair of ankle injuries to the deltoid ligament. Foot Ankle Clin 1999;4(4):745–53.
65. Lamm BM, Mendicino RW, Catanzariti AR, et al. Static rearfoot alignment: a comparison of clinical and radiographic measures. J Am Podiatr Med Assoc 2005;95:26–33.
66. Gill JB, Risko T, Raducan J, et al. Comparison of manual and gravity stress radiographs for the evaluation of supination-external rotation fibular fractures. J Bone Joint Surg Am 2007;89:994–9.
67. Chen PY, Wang TG, Wang CL. Ultrasonographic examination of the deltoid ligament in bimalleolar equivalent fractures. Foot Ankle Int 2008;29(9):883–6.
68. Henari S, Banks LN, Radiovanovic I, et al. Ultrasonography as a diagnostic tool in assessing deltoid ligament injury in supination external rotation fractures of the ankle. Orthopedics 2011;34(10):e639–43.
69. Chhabra A, Subhawong TK, Carrino JA. MR imaging of deltoid ligament pathologic findings and associated impingement syndromes. Radiographics 2010; 30(3):751–61.
70. Boyer MI, Bowen V, Weiler P. Reconstruction of a severe grinding injury to the medial malleolus and the deltoid ligament of the ankle using a free plantaris tendon graft and vascularized gracilis free muscle transfer: a case report. J Trauma 1994;36:454–7.
71. Hintermann B, Valderrabano V, Kundert HP. Lengthening of the lateral column and reconstruction of the medial soft tissue for treatment of acquired flatfoot deformity associated with insufficiency of the posterior tibial tendon. Foot Ankle Int 1999;20:622–99.
72. Deland JT, de Asla RJ, Segal A. Reconstruction of the chronically failed deltoid ligament: a new technique. Foot Ankle Int 2004;25(11):795–9.
73. Ellis SJ, Williams BR, Wagshul AD, et al. Deltoid ligament reconstruction with peroneus longus autograft in flatfoot deformity. Foot Ankle Int 2010;31(9):781–9.
74. Kelkian H, Kelkian A. Disruptions of the deltoid ligament. In: Kelkian H, Kelkian A, editors. Disorders of the ankle. Philadelphia: WB Saunders; 1985. p. 339–70.
75. Leach RE, Schepsis AA. Acute injuries to ligaments of the ankle. In: Ecarts CM, editor. Surgery of the musculoskeletal system, vol. 4. New York: Churchill Livingstone; 1990. p. 3887–913.
76. Wiltberger BR, Mallory TM. A new method for the reconstruction of the deltoid ligament of the ankle. Orthop Rev 1972;1:37–41.
77. Jeng CL, Bluman EM, Myerson MS. Minimally invasive deltoid ligament reconstruction for Stage IV flatfoot deformity. Foot Ankle Int 2011;32(1):21–30.
78. Kitaoka HB, Luo ZP, An KN. Reconstruction operations for acquired flatfoot: biomechanical evaluation. Foot Ankle Int 1998;19:203–7.
79. Haddad SL, Dedhia S, Ren Y, et al. Deltoid ligament reconstruction: a novel technique with biomechanical analysis. Foot Ankle Int 2010;31(7):639–51.
80. Bluman EM, Khazen G, Haraguchi N, et al. Minimally invasive deltoid reconstruction: a comparison of three techniques. Presented at the Proceedings of the 36th Annual Winter Meeting. Speciality Day AOFAS. Chicago, March 25, 2006.
81. Myerson M. Adult acquired flatfoot deformity. Treatment of dysfunction of the posterior tibial tendon. J Bone Joint Surg Am 1996;78:780–92.

82. Egol KA, Parisien JS. Impingement syndrome of the ankle caused by a medial meniscoid lesion. Arthroscopy 1997;13(4):522–5.
83. Mosier-La Clair SM, Monroe MT. Medial impingement syndrome of the anterior tibiotalar fascicle of the deltoid ligament on the talus. Foot Ankle Int 2000; 21(5):385–91.
84. Umans H. Ankle impingement syndromes. Semin Musculoskelet Radiol 2002;6: 133–9.
85. Robinson P, White LM. Soft-tissue and osseous impingement syndromes of the ankle: role of imaging in diagnosis and management. Radiographics 2002;22: 1457–69.
86. Robinson P, White LM, Salonen D, et al. Anteromedial impingement of the ankle: using MR arthrography to assess the anteromedial recess. AJR Am J Roentgenol 2002;178:601–4.
87. Jowett AJ, Birks CL, Blackney MC. Medial malleolar stress fracture secondary to chronic ankle impingement. Foot Ankle Int 2008;29(7):716–21.
88. Paterson RS, Brown JN, Roberts SN. The posteromedial impingement lesion of the ankle: a series of six cases. Am J Sports Med 2001;29:550–7.
89. Coral A. The radiology of skeletal elements in the subtibial region: incidence and significance. Skeletal Radiol 1987;16:298–303.
90. Holle F. Über ide inkonstanstanten Elemente am menschlichen Fussskelett [Inaugural dissertation]. Munich, 1938.
91. Powell HD. Extra centre of ossification for the medial malleolus in children. J Bone Joint Surg Br 1961;43(1):107–13.
92. Silver RL, Garza J, Rang M. The myth of muscle balance: a study of relative strengths and excursions of normal muscles about the foot and ankle. J Bone Joint Surg Br 1985;67:432–7.
93. Wickiewicz TL, Roy RR, Powell PL, et al. Muscle: architecture of the lower limb. Clin Orthop Relat Res 1983;179:275–83.
94. Van Dijk CN, Kort N, Scholten PE. Tendoscopy of the posterior tibial tendon. Arthroscopy 1997;1:471–8.
95. Frey C, Shereff M, Greenidge N. Vascularity of the posterior tibial tendon. J Bone Joint Surg Am 1990;72:884–8.
96. Bloome DM, Marymont JV, Varner KE. Variations on the insertion of the posterior tibialis tendon: a cadaveric study. Foot Ankle Int 2003;24(10):780–3.
97. Brodsky JW. Preliminary gait analysis results after posterior tibial tendon reconstruction. Foot Ankle Int 2004;25(2):96–100.
98. Johnson KA, Strom DE. Tibialis posterior tendon dysfunction. Clin Orthop 1989; 239:196–206.
99. Myerson MS. Adult acquired flatfoot deformity: treatment of dysfunction of the posterior tibial tendon. Instr Course Lect 1997;46:393–405.
100. Myerson M, Solomon G, Shereff M. Posterior tibial dysfunction: its association with seronegative inflammatory disease. Foot Ankle Int 1989;9:219–25.
101. Supple KM, Hanft JR, Murphy BJ, et al. Posterior tibial tendon dysfunction. Semin Arthritis Rheum 1992;22:106–13.
102. Bare AA, Haddad SL. Tenosynovitis of the posterior tibial tendon. Foot Ankle Clin 2001;6(1):37–66.
103. Trevino S, Gould N, Korson R. Surgical treatment of stenosing tenosynovitis at the ankle. Foot Ankle 1981;2:37–45.
104. Cooper AJ, Mizel MS, Patel PD, et al. Comparison of MRI and local anesthetic tendon sheath injection in the diagnosis of posterior tibial tendon tenosynovitis. Foot Ankle Int 2007;28(11):1124–7.

105. Alexander J, Johnson KA, Berquist TH. Magnetic imaging in the diagnosis of disruption of the posterior tibial tendon. Foot Ankle Int 1987;8:144–7.
106. Miller SD, Van Holsbeeck M, Boruta PM, et al. Ultrasound in the diagnosis of posterior tibial tendon pathology. Foot Ankle Int 1996;17:555–8.
107. Chen Y, Liang S. Diagnostic efficacy of ultrasonography in stage 1 posterior tibial tendon dysfunction: sonographic-surgical correlation. J Ultrasound Med 1997;16:417–23.
108. Alvarez RG, Marini A, Schmitt C, et al. Stage I and II posterior tibial dysfunction treated by a structured nonoperative management protocol: an orthosis and exercise program. Foot Ankle Int 2006;27(1):2–8.
109. Giza E, Cush G, Schon LC. The flexible flatfoot in the adult. Foot Ankle Clin 2007; 12:251–71.
110. Holmes GB, Mann RA. Possible epidemiological factors associated with rupture of the posterior tibial tendon. Foot Ankle 1992;13:70–9.
111. Chauveaux D, Souilaac V, Laffenetre O, et al. Contribution of tendinoscopy in ankle tendon disease: preliminary analysis of 22 cases. J Bone Joint Surg Br 2005;87(Suppl II):114.
112. Chow HT, Chan KB, Lui TH. Tendoscopic debridement for stage I posterior tibial tendon dysfunction. Knee Surg Sports Traumatol Arthrosc 2005;13(8):695–8.
113. Porter DA, Baxter DE, Clanton TO, et al. Posterior tibial tendon tears in young competitive athletes: two case reports. Foot Ankle Int 1998;19(9):627–30.
114. Marks RM, Schon LC. Post-traumatic posterior tibialis insertional elongation with functional incompetency: a case report. Foot Ankle Int 1998;19(3):180–3.
115. Needleman RL. A surgical approach for flexible flatfeet in adults including a subtalar arthroereisis with the MBA subtalar implant. Foot Ankle Int 2006; 27(1):9–18.
116. VanAman S, Schon L. Subtalar arthroereisis as adjunct treatment for type II posterior tibial tendon deficiency. Tech Foot Ankle Surg 2006;5(2):117–25.
117. Gluck GS, Heckman DS, Parekh SG. Tendon disorders of the foot and ankle, part 3: the posterior tibial tendon. Am J Sports Med 2010;38(10):2133–44.
118. Masterson E, Jagannathan S, Borton D, et al. Pes planus in childhood due to tibialis posterior tendon injuries. Treatment by flexor hallucis tendon transfer. J Bone Joint Surg Br 1994;76(3):444–6.
119. Penney KE, Wiener BD, Magill RM. Traumatic rupture of the tibialis posterior tendon after ankle fracture: a case report. Am J Orthop 2000;29(1):41–3.
120. Uzel AP, Massicot R, Delattre O, et al. Traumatic rupture of the tibialis posterior tendon after ankle fracture: three cases and a review of the literature. Rev Chir Orthop Reparatrice Appar Mot 2006;92(3):283–9.
121. Ceccarelli F, Faldini C, Pagkrati S, et al. Rupture of the tibialis posterior tendon in a closed ankle fracture: a case report. Chir Organi Mov 2008;91(3):167–70.
122. West MA, Sangani C, Toh E. Tibialis posterior tendon rupture associated with a closed medial malleolar fracture: a case report and review of the literature. J Foot Ankle Surg 2010;49(6):565.e9–12.
123. Akra GA, Saeed KK, Limaye RV. An unusual etiology for adult-acquired flatfoot. J Foot Ankle Surg 2010;49(5):488.e11–4.
124. Henceroth WD II, Deyerle WM. The acquired unilateral flatfoot in the adult: some causative factors. Foot Ankle 1982;2:304–8.
125. Kettlekamp DB, Alexander HH. Spontaneous rupture of the posterior tibial tendon. J Bone Joint Surg Am 1969;51:759–64.
126. Woods L, Leach RE. Posterior tibial tendon rupture in athletic people. Am J Sports Med 1991;19(5):495–8.

127. Marcus RE, Goodfellow DB, Pfister ME. The difficult diagnosis of posterior tibialis tendon rupture in sports injuries. Orthopedics 1995;18(8):715–21.
128. Martius C. Notes sur un cas de luxation du muscle tibial posterieur, etc. Bull R Med Belg 1874;4:103.
129. Nava BE. Traumatic dislocation of the tibialis posterior tendon at the ankle: a report of a case. J Bone Joint Surg Br 1968;50:150–1.
130. Walker RH, Farris C. Irreducible fracture-dislocations of the ankle associated with interposition of the tibialis posterior tendon. Clin Orthop Relat Res 1981; 160:212–6.
131. Søballe K, Kjaersgaard-Andersen P. Ruptured tibialis posterior tendon in a closed ankle fracture. Clin Orthop Relat Res 1988;231:140–3.
132. Ermis MN, Yagmurlu MF, Kilinc AS, et al. Irreducible fracture dislocation of the ankle caused by tibialis posterior tendon interposition. J Foot Ankle Surg 2010;49(2):166–71.
133. Mitchell K, Mencia MM, Hoford R. Tibialis posterior dislocation: a case report. Foot (Edinb) 2011;21(3):154–6.
134. Boss AP, Hintermann B. Tibialis posterior dislocation in combination with Achilles tendon rupture: a case report. Foot Ankle Int 2008;29(6):633–6.
135. Langan P, Weiss CA. Dislocation of the tibialis posterior, a complication of tarsal tunnel decompression: a case report. Clin Orthop 1980;146:226–7.
136. Lohrer H, Nauck T. Posterior tibial tendon dislocation: a systematic review of the literature and presentation of a case. Br J Sports Med 2010;44(6): 398–406.
137. Loncarich DP, Clapper M. Dislocation of posterior tibial tendon. Foot Ankle Int 1998;19(12):821–4.
138. Vilas O, Montojo R, Sorroche P. Traumatic dislocation of tibialis posterior tendon: a case report in a Tae-Kwon-Do athlete. Clin J Sport Med 2009;19(1):68–9.
139. Deland JT, Hamilton WG. Posterior tibial tendon tears in dancers. Clin Sports Med 2008;27:289–94.
140. Soler RR, Gallart Castany FJ, Riba Ferret J, et al. Traumatic dislocation of the tibialis posterior tendon at the ankle level. J Trauma 1986;26(11):1049–52.
141. Bencardino J, Rosenberg ZS, Beltran J, et al. MR imaging if dislocation of the posterior tibial tendon. AJR Am J Roentgenol 1997;169(4):1109–12.
142. Ouzounian TJ, Myerson MS. Dislocation of the posterior tibial tendon. Foot Ankle Int 1992;13:215–9.
143. Coskun N, Yuksel M, Cevner M, et al. Incidence of accessory ossicles and sesamoid bones in the feet: a radiographic study of the Turkish subjects. Surg Radiol Anat 2009;31(1):19–24.
144. Bizarro AH. On the traumatology of the sesamoid structures. Ann Surg 1921;74: 783–91.
145. Grogan D, Gasser S, Ogden J. The painful accessory navicular: a clinical and histopathological study. Foot Ankle 1989;10:164–9.
146. Geist ES. The accessory scaphoid bone. J Bone Joint Surg Am 1925;7:570–4.
147. Dwight T. Variations of the bones of the hands and feet: a clinical atlas. Philadelphia: JB Lippincott; 1907.
148. Sella E, Lawson E. Biomechanics of the accessory navicular synchondrosis. Foot Ankle 1987;8:156–63.
149. Ray S, Goldberg VM. Surgical treatment of the accessory navicular. Clin Orthop 1983;177:61–6.
150. Lawson JP. Symptomatic radiographic variants in extremities. Radiology 1985; 157:625.

151. Lepore L, Francobandiera C, Maffulli N. Fracture of the os tibiale externum in a decathlete. J Foot Surg 1990;29:366–8.
152. Wong MW, Griffith JF. Magnetic imaging in adolescent painful flexible flatfoot. Foot Ankle Int 2009;30(4):303–8.
153. Chuang YW, Tsai WS, Chen KH, et al. Clinical use of high-resolution ultrasonography for the diagnosis of type II accessory navicular bone. Am J Phys Med Rehabil 2012;91(2):177–81.
154. Biersack HJ, Wingenfeld C, Hinterthaner B, et al. SPECT-CT of the foot. Nuklearmedizin 2012;51(1):26–31.
155. Leonard ZC, Fortin PT. Adolescent accessory navicular. Foot Ankle Clin 2010; 15(2):337–47.
156. Jasiewicz B, Potacczek T, Kacki W, et al. Results of simple excision technique in the surgical treatment of symptomatic accessory navicular bones. Foot Ankle Surg 2008;14:57–61.
157. Micheli LJ, Nielson JH, Ascani C, et al. Treatment of painful accessory navicular: a modification to a simple excision. Foot Ankle Spec 2008;1:214–7.
158. Senses I, Kiler E, Gunai I. Restoring the continuity of the tibialis posterior tendon in the treatment of symptomatic accessory navicular with flat feet. J Orthop Sci 2004;9:408–9.
159. Kidner FC. The pre-hallux (accessory scaphoid) in its relation to the flat-foot. J Bone Joint Surg Am 1929;11:831–7.
160. Kidner FC. The prehallux in relation to flat-foot. J Am Med Assoc 1933;101(20): 1539–42.
161. Veitch JM. Evaluation of the Kidner procedure in treatment of symptomatic accessory tarsal scaphoid. Clin Orthop 1978;131:210–3.
162. Nakayama S, Sugimoto K, Takakura Y, et al. Percutaneous drilling of symptomatic accessory navicular in young athletes. Am J Sports Med 2005;33(4):531–5.
163. Chung JW, Chu IT. Outcome of fusion of a painful accessory navicular to the primary navicular. Foot Ankle Int 2009;30(2):106–9.
164. Malicky ES, Levine DS, Sangeorzan BJ. Modification of the Kidner procedure with fusion of the primary and accessory navicular bones. Foot Ankle Int 1999;20:53–4.
165. Scott AT, Abesan VJ, Saluta JR, et al. Fusion versus excision of the symptomatic type II accessory navicular: a prospective study. Foot Ankle Int 2009;30:10–5.

Treatment of Recurring Peroneal Tendon Subluxation in Athletes
Endoscopic Repair of the Retinaculum

Stephane Guillo, MD[a],*,
James D.F. Calder, TD, MD, FRCS(Tr & Orth), FFSEM(UK)[b,c]

KEYWORDS

- Endoscopy • Peroneal tendon • Peroneal dislocation • Tendoscopy

KEY POINTS

- Peroneal tendon subluxation is a rare lesion that must be considered in the event of ankle trauma.
- Chronic subluxation in athletes require surgical stabilization.
- The superior retinaculum may be repaired by endoscopy, giving good short- and medium-term results.

INTRODUCTION

Traumatic peroneal tendon subluxation is a rare lesion mainly affecting young adults. This lesion occurs most frequently during sporting activities and generally during an ankle sprain. There is consensus regarding the need for surgical stabilization in symptomatic patients, but there is also general agreement that acute subluxation or dislocations may require surgery in the athlete.

Many surgical techniques have been described to treat this lesion. They fall into 3 main categories: tendon rerouting using the calcaneofibular ligament to replace the incompetent superior retinaculum,[1–4] retinacular reconstruction or reinforcement[5–10] and retromalleolar groove deepening.[11–15] Overall, the studies reported excellent or good results in 90% of cases, although the number of patients was frequently low. There have been reports of significant complications following open surgical procedures (infection, wound problems, bone block fracture, permanent discomfort, recurrent subluxation and skin hypersensitivity), but overall the results of surgery have been considered good, with a high rate of return to sporting activities.

a Centre for Orthopaedic Sports Surgery, 2 rue Negrevergne, Bordeaux-Mérignac 33700, France; b Department of Orthopaedics, Chelsea and Westminster Hospital, 369 Fulham Road, London SW10 9NH, United Kingdom; c The Fortius Clinic, 17 Fitzhardinge Street, London W1H 6EQ, United Kingdom
* Corresponding author.
E-mail address: docteurguillochirurgien@gmail.com

Foot Ankle Clin N Am 18 (2013) 293–300
http://dx.doi.org/10.1016/j.fcl.2013.02.007
1083-7515/13/$ – see front matter © 2013 Elsevier Inc. All rights reserved.

foot.theclinics.com

Das De and Balasubramaniam[6] suggested the stripped retinacular pocket was similar to the Bankart lesion of the shoulder. They described a direct repair using sutures to reattach the superior peroneal retinaculum (SPR) to the fibula and termed it the Singapore operation. Hui and colleagues[16] reported on the long-term results of 21 cases. There were no recurrences, and 18 out of 21 patients had good or excellent results. In 2006, Adachi and colleagues[17] reported the results of 18 cases of SPR reattachment using a tissue tensioner device to optimize retinacular tension. At 2 years, all had returned to their preinjury level of activity with no recurrences.

There are several published methods combining direct repair of the SPR with deepening of the fibula groove. Zoellner and Clancy[13] described a simple technique of deepening the groove by local excision of bone and excavation. Twelve consecutive cases were reviewed by Kollias and Ferkel,[14] with no recurrences at 8 months, and 91% returning to full activity. Karlsson and colleagues[15] presented the results of 15 patients at 3.5 years treated by deepening the groove with a curved chisel and repair of the retinaculum. There were no recurrences and good or excellent results in 87% of cases, with 13% of cases having fair results due to postoperative stiffness and pain on exertion. Porter and colleagues[19] described a modification of this technique with recession of the posterior cortex and repair of the SPR in 14 patients. Rather than employing standard postoperative cast immobilization, a walker boot was used with physiotherapy starting at 1 week postoperatively. At 3 years, there were no recurrences, minimal postoperative symptoms, and an average return to sports of 3 months.

Conventional open surgery inevitably requires the sectioning of the stabilizing structures that are to be repaired; therefore the development of an endoscopic technique to reproduce the same results as the open procedure is an attractive alternative. Few cases have been published; 2 techniques have been described. The first consists of deepening the groove,[20] and the second consists of reinserting the peroneal tendon sheath.[18] This article presents the technique of 1 of the authors (SG), using anchors, inspired by the arthroscopic repair of Bankart shoulder lesions and the subsequent reports of open SPR reattachment described previously.

ANATOMY

The shape of the posterior surface of the lateral malleolus appears to play an important role in stability. In 8 out of 10 dissections, there is a genuine groove in this region.[1,21,22] The absence of a bone groove or even a convex surface increases the risk of tendon instability.

The SPR originates on the posterolateral surface of the fibula, passing over the tendons and attaching to the lateral surface of the calcaneus (**Fig. 1**). It plays a major role in stabilizing the peroneal tendons. Isolating sections of the SPR causes subluxation when the foot is pronated.[23]

It is important to note that there is no solid anchor point on the bone ridge limiting the lateral extent of the retromalleolar groove. The SPR attaches to the lateral malleolar periosteum. Therefore, during peroneal tendon subluxation, the SPR is only rarely torn but rather lifted from the fibula along with the lateral malleolar periosteum in a single piece.[24] This then leaves a pocket on the lateral aspect of the fibula into which the tendons may recurrently sublux.

SURGICAL TECHNIQUE
Instruments

Some surgeons have described using a 2.7 mm arthroscope for tendinoscopy.[25,26] The authors prefer, like others,[24] to use a standard 4 mm arthroscope, as this has

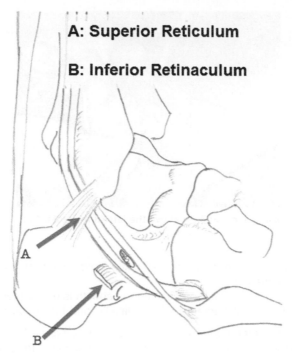

A: Superior Reticulum

B: Inferior Retinaculum

Fig. 1. Anatomy of the retinaculum.

the advantage of a broader field of vision and increased fluid flow. A low-pressure gravity flow of fluid is recommended to avoid fluid extravasation. The authors recommend the use of a 3.5 to 4 mm shave blade, to reduce the risk of iatrogenic tendon trauma.

The authors prefer to use a number 15 scalpel blade, as it is safer and less traumatic than a number 11 blade, and the authors also recommend the creation of an initial approach using 2 small Gillis hooks. Furthermore, a small curved Halstead forceps is essential. This instrument avoids causing trauma to subcutaneous nerves after incising the skin.

Patient Positioning

The procedure may be performed under general or regional anesthesia with an above the knee tourniquet. Instead of the supine position, with a cushion placed under the prone buttock,[20,27] the authors prefer the lateral position. Care must always be taken to place the arthroscopic tower in front of the patient, at the level of the operated foot, the surgeon positioning himself or herself behind.

Approach

Two incisions are made, one 3 cm proximal and the other 3 cm distal to the lateral malleolus. Several authors[16,22,24] have described the first incision being made distally. The authors recommend first creating the proximal incision for several reasons (**Fig. 2**):

- Locating the peroneal tendon sheath is much easier from this position, as it is thicker here.

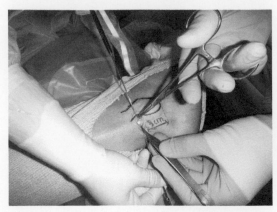

Fig. 2. The first proximal incision 3 cm above the lateral malleolar tip.

- The sural nerve is further toward the midline more proximally and therefore less likely to be damaged.
- Progressing distally in the peroneal tendon sheath is easier than moving proximally; the sheath wall becomes thinner distally, and the space is less confined.

Using the Gillis hook retractors, and under direct vision, expose the peroneal tendon sheath and make a longitudinal incision. It is then easy to insert the blunt arthroscopy trocar into the sheath.

Push the arthroscope distally, beyond the tip of the malleolus. The position of the second approach can then be determined using a needle. Transillumination is used to avoid the sural nerve (**Fig. 3**).

An inspection of the tendons can then begin distally with each tendon within its own sheath, up to the retromalleolar groove in the fibula. This inspection provides a view of virtually the whole region.

The probe is inserted to assess for concomitant lesions such as tears. The tendons, sheath, and separation pocket can be readily examined (**Fig. 4**). The arthroscope and shaver portals may be interchanged. Inspection usually reveals a separate pocket

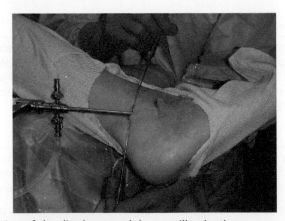

Fig. 3. Identification of the distal approach by transillumination.

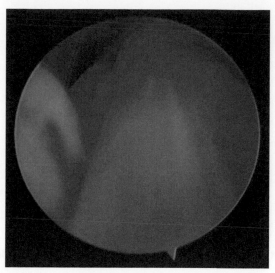

Fig. 4. Exploration of the peroneal tendon sheath.

around the lateral margin of the fibula in continuity with the periosteum and retinaculum, generally accompanied by a fissuring or tendinopathy of the peroneus brevis at the same level. Fibrous debris may be debrided with the 3.5 mm shaver to improve vision. The shaver is then used to roughen the lateral aspect of the fibula to prepare the surface for reattachment of the SPR (a burr is too aggressive for this purpose) (**Fig. 5**). The SPR is then reattached and tensioned to the fibula using 2 JuggerKnot 1.8 bone anchors (Biomet). The correct site for the anchor is identified with a needle, and a 5 mm incision is made, through which the anchor is inserted. The main difficulty at this point is in passing the anchor thread through the retinaculum at the desired location to allow a tensioning effect of the retinacular complex (**Fig. 6**).

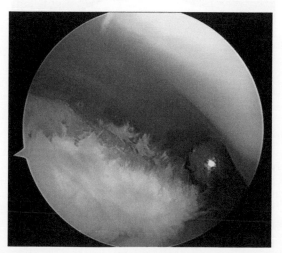

Fig. 5. Preparation of the lateral border of the fibula.

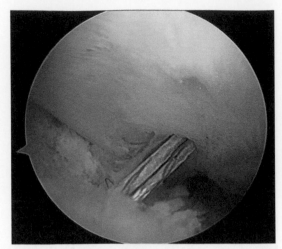

Fig. 6. Jogger knot 1.8 (Biomet) positioned at the top of the lateral malleolus.

A large-gauge needle onto which a shuttle relay has been looped (single-strand, of sufficient diameter to withstand traction, generally 2/0) is used to thread through the SPR (**Fig. 7**).

Four passes are made (2 threads per anchor), and the sutures are tightened, reattaching the SPR to the fibula (**Fig. 8**). Skin closure is then performed.

For postoperative care, the authors recommend 6 weeks of immobilization during which no weight should be placed on the ankle and after which ankle range-of-motion and proprioception/strengthening techniques are initiated.

PRELIMINARY RESULTS

Seven patients have been operated on to date, all men. The mean age at the time of operation was of 33.1 years (19–46 years). Five patients practiced a sport at a

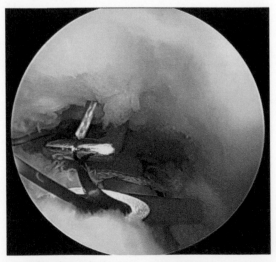

Fig. 7. Shuttle relay passing through the SPR.

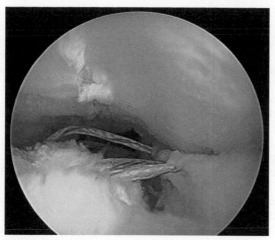

Fig. 8. Tightening of the suture repair.

competitive level (1 skiing, 2 rugby, and 2 soccer). In all cases, the hind foot was normally aligned. In 6 cases, the mechanism of injury was an ankle inversion/supination sprain, and in 1 case, a skiing-related trauma. Average follow-up was 21.8 months (range 15–28 months). No relapse occurred. All patients were able to resume their normal activities and sports activities at the same level. One patient presented with skin irritation caused by the suture knot under the skin and requiring repeat surgery to remove the thread after 3 months.

SUMMARY

Among the range of available techniques, endoscopic retinacular repair is attractive in that it preserves the anatomy as much as possible. The initial results are encouraging with no early complications, and the technique allows patients to return to sporting activities. Long-term studies involving a larger number of cases will, however, be required to demonstrate the efficacy of this technique.

REFERENCES

1. Poll RG, Duijfjes F. The treatment of recurrent dislocation of the peroneal tendons. J Bone Joint Surg Br 1984;66(1):98–100.
2. Sarmiento A, Wolf M. Subluxation of peroneal tendons. Case treated by rerouting tendons under calcaneofibular ligament. J Bone Joint Surg Am 1975;57(1):115–6.
3. Martens MA, Noyez JF, Mulier JC. Recurrent dislocation of the peroneal tendons. Results of rerouting the tendons under the calcaneofibular ligament. Am J Sports Med 1986;14(2):148–50.
4. Pozo JL, Jackson AM. A rerouting operation for dislocation of peroneal tendons: operative technique and case report. Foot Ankle 1984;5(1):42–4.
5. Alm A, Lamke LO, Liljedahl SO. Surgical treatment of dislocation of the peroneal tendons. Injury 1975;7(1):14–9.
6. Das De S, Balasubramaniam P. A repair operation for recurrent dislocation of peroneal tendons. J Bone Joint Surg Br 1985;67(4):585–7.
7. Tourne Y, Saragaglia D, Benzakour D, et al. Traumatic luxation of the peroneal tendons. Report of 36 cases. Int Orthop 1995;19(4):197–203 [in French].

8. Thomas JL, Sheridan L, Graviet S. A modification of the Ellis Jones procedure for chronic peroneal subsubluxation. J Foot Surg 1992;31(5):454–8.
9. Escalas F, Figueras JM, Merino JA. Dislocation of the peroneal tendons. Long-term results of surgical treatment. J Bone Joint Surg Am 1980;62(3):451–3.
10. Jones EB. Operative treatment of chronic dislocation of the peroneal tendons. J Bone Joint Surg 1932;14:574.
11. Marti R. Dislocation of the peroneal tendons. Am J Sports Med 1977;5(1):19–22.
12. Larsen E, Flink-Olsen M, Seerup K. Surgery for recurrent dislocation of the peroneal tendons. Acta Orthop Scand 1984;55(5):554–5.
13. Zoellner G, Clancy W Jr. Recurrent dislocation of the peroneal tendon. J Bone Joint Surg Am 1979;61(2):292–4.
14. Kollias SL, Ferkel RD. Fibular grooving for recurrent peroneal tendon subluxation. Am J Sports Med 1997;25(3):329–35.
15. Karlsson J, Eriksson BI, Sward L. Recurrent dislocation of the peroneal tendons. Scand J Med Sci Sports 1996;6(4):242–6.
16. Hui JH, Das De S, Balasubramaniam P. The Singapore operation for recurrent dislocation of peroneal tendons: long-term results. J Bone Joint Surg Br 1998; 80(2):325–7.
17. Adachi N, Fukuhara K, Tanaka H, et al. Superior retinaculoplasty for recurrent dislocation of peroneal tendons. Foot Ankle Int 2006;27(12):1074–8.
18. Lui TH. Endoscopic peroneal retinaculum reconstruction. Knee Surg Sports Traumatol Arthrosc 2006;14(5):478–81.
19. Porter D, McCarroll J, Knapp E, et al. Peroneal tendon subluxation in athletes: fibular groove deepening and retinacular reconstruction. Foot Ankle Int 2005; 26(6):436–41.
20. van Dijk CN, Kort N. Tendoscopy of the peroneal tendons. Arthroscopy 1998; 14(5):471–8.
21. Edwards M. The relation of the peroneal tendons to the fibula, calacaneus and cuboieum. Am J Anat 1929;42:213.
22. Mabit C, Salanne P, Boncoeur-Martel M, et al. La gouttière rétromalléolaire latérale: étude radio-anatomique. Bull Assoc Anat (Nancy) 1996;80(249):17–21.
23. Purnell ML, Drummond DS, Engber WD, et al. Congenital dislocation of the peroneal tendons in the calcaneovalgus foot. J Bone Joint Surg Br 1983;65(3):316–9.
24. Eckert WR, Davis EA Jr. Acute rupture of the peroneal retinaculum. J Bone Joint Surg Am 1976;58(5):670–2.
25. Sammarco VJ. Peroneal tendoscopy: indications and techniques. Sports Med Arthrosc 2009;17(2):94–9.
26. Scholten PE, van Dijk CN. Tendoscopy of the peroneal tendons. Foot Ankle Clin 2006;11(2):415–20, vii.
27. Laffenêtre O, Villet L, Solofomalala D, et al. Tendinoscopie de l'arrière pied. In: Leemrijse T, Valtin B, editors. Pathologie du pied et de la cheville. Paris (France): Masson; 2009. p. 522.

Posterior Ankle Impingement in Dancers and Athletes

Andrew J. Roche, MSc, FRCS (Tr & Orth)[a],*,
James D.F. Calder, TD, MD, FRCS (Tr & Orth), FFSEM (UK)[a,b],
R. Lloyd Williams, FRCS (Tr & Orth)[c]

KEYWORDS

• Posterior • Ankle • Impingement • Arthroscopy • Athlete

KEY POINTS

- Magnetic resonance imaging (MRI) is the gold standard radiological investigation for posterior ankle impingement. The clinician should also remember that computed tomography is still useful, even in conjunction with MRI to recognize smaller bony impingement lesions or avulsion fragments.
- In the athlete, targeted, ultrasound-guided, interim local anesthetic and steroid injections for posterior ankle impingement lesions can produce rapid symptom relief and enable a player to complete a season.
- Posterior arthroscopic surgical excision is recommended to ensure rapid return to full sporting activity. Open excision is an option, but the athlete's time to return to sport is delayed.
- Posteromedial ankle impingement should be considered in a patient with a history of anterolateral ligament injury and ruled out with careful examination and investigations.

The origins of posterior ankle impingement (PAI) are multifactorial. It is a term used to encompass any disease that is characterized by increasing pain or discomfort, usually exacerbated while adopting a plantarflexed posture of the ankle. As many surgeons and therapists understand, it is rarely found to be a significant problem in the nonathlete or in athletes who are infrequently required to forcibly plantarflex the ankle joint, but it can be seen to be a severely debilitating problem for recreational or competitive athletes. The reason why those often afflicted are involved in recurrent plantarflexion movement is usually simple biomechanics; for example, ballet dancers (especially when adopting the positions of en pointe (**Fig. 1**) or demi-pointe), runners and field athletes (often at the terminal stance phase), and soccer players (either running with sudden changes of direction or at the moment of ball strike on the forefoot).

The normal (and normal variant) bony and soft tissue anatomy of the posterior ankle and hindfoot along with overuse of the region both contribute to the development of

The authors have nothing to disclose.
[a] Chelsea and Westminster Hospital NHS Foundation Trust, 369 Fulham Road, London SW10 9NH, UK; [b] The Fortius Clinic, 17 Fitzhardinge Street, London W1H 6EQ, UK; [c] The London Orthopaedic Clinic, 79 Wimpole Street, London W1G 9RY, UK
* Corresponding author.
E-mail address: andrew.roche@me.com

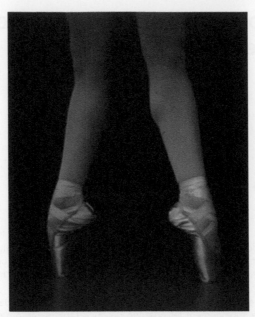

Fig. 1. Ballet dancer en pointe.

posterior impingement. It is important, through accurate clinical examination and appropriate imaging studies, that the clinician identifies the cause of the condition, because more and more conditions are being recognized. The necessary treatment can then be guided by these findings to enable a rapid and safe return to function for a patient who is often a high-level or high-demand athlete keen to resume normal activity as quickly as possible.

ANATOMY

A thorough understanding of the anatomy and its subtle variations is vital to appreciate this condition. The important structures can be broadly separated into osseous and soft tissue structures.

Bony Anatomy

The osseous contributions to PAI are the distal tibial slope, the superior aspect of the calcaneum, and the interposed posterior talus. The talocrural or ankle joint develops as a synovial hinge or ginglymoid joint to allow functional dorsi and plantar flexion with a slightly oblique axis of motion. The normal range of motion in an adult population varies between 20° dorsiflexion and 50° plantarflexion.[1] In ballet dancers, the range of plantarflexion at the ankle joint has been reported to be more than 100°[2] by goniometer measurements. However, this method only crudely measures the relationship of the foot with the tibia and does not account for contributions for plantarflexion occurring distal to the ankle joint, which may increase the appearance of ankle joint motion (ie, tarsometatarsal motion in the sagittal plane). Recent studies using radiographs to analyze motion in the foot and ankle during positions of extreme plantar and dorsiflexion in female ballet dancers found that ankle joint plantarflexion in 7 dancers was 57°.[3] This overall increased range of motion helps achieve en pointe and demi-pointe positioning in classical ballet dancers. In some cases, ballerinas with reduced range of plantarflexion can invert their foot with the heel, adopting a varus position (sickling-in) in an attempt to achieve increased height in en pointe positioning. This position can produce excess strain and attrition on the lateral ligament complex and predispose to injury.

The posterior talus typically develops with 2 posterior processes or tubercles (a medial and lateral tubercle), between which lies a groove for the flexor hallucis longus (FHL) tendon (**Fig. 2**).

The talus originally develops from a primary ossific nucleus; however, between the ages of 8 and 11 years, a smaller secondary ossification center arises posterior to the lateral tubercle. In 85%, it fuses with the posterolateral tubercle within 12 months of its appearance, and in the remainder, it persists as an unfused ossicle. This condition is known as an os trigonum (**Fig. 3**). An os trigonum can appear in up to 25% of the normal adult population on radiographs.[4] In cases in which the posterolateral process of the talus projects more posteriorly than normal, it is referred to as a Stieda process (**Fig. 4**).[5]

The superior aspect of the calcaneus can contribute to PAI. Prominence of the posterior superolateral surface of the calcaneum has, in the past, been referred to as a Haglund deformity (**Fig. 5**). This is often a confusing term to use for this condition, and a more accurate description has recently been adopted, referring to the nature of the soft tissue lesion in association with any prominence encountered on calcaneus.[6] Although it is more likely to cause Achilles tendon problems or retrocalcaneal bursitis, it should be considered as a potential cause of PAI. The presence of a prominent calcaneal tuberosity was evident in 64% of ballet dancers on magnetic resonance imaging (MRI) scan in an anatomic study, which could be assumed to be a likely contributing factor to PAI.[7]

In the same anatomic study, it was evident that the shape of the posterior tibial slope may contribute to the symptoms. A significantly downward sloping posterior tibial lip was discovered in 25% of dancers and, because of the simple biomechanics of bony impingement in plantarflexion, this should also be considered an important bony source of PAI (**Fig. 6**).

Soft Tissue Anatomy

The bony anatomy and restricted space in the posterior recesses of the ankle and subtalar joints do not accommodate abundant soft tissues well, especially in the positions

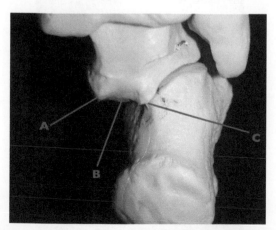

Fig. 2. The posterior aspect of the Talus. A, posteromedial tubercle; B, groove for FHL; C, posterior tubercle.

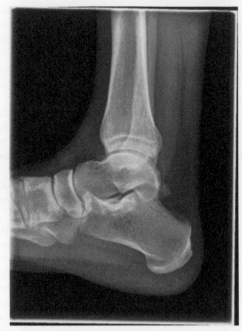

Fig. 3. Lateral radiograph showing an os trigonum.

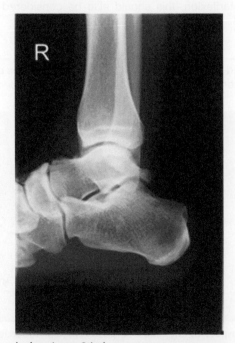

Fig. 4. Lateral radiograph showing a Stieda process.

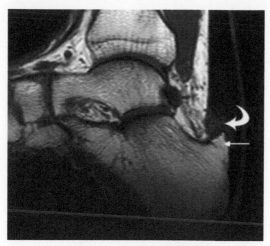

Fig. 5. A posterosuperior prominence (*straight arrow*) in association with insertional Achilles tendinopathy (*curved arrow*).

of extreme plantarflexion adopted by many athletes. For this reason, the normal anatomic soft tissue structures of the posterior ankle can easily contribute to the onset of PAI. The soft tissue structures of importance include the synovial capsule of the ankle and subtalar joints, the FHL tendon, and the ligaments of the posterior ankle.

The posterior ankle ligaments include the posterior inferior tibiofibular ligament (PITFL), the intermalleolar or transverse tibiofibular ligament, the tibial slip ligament, and the posterior talofibular ligament (PTFL) **(Fig. 7)**.

Intimate knowledge of the anatomic locations of these structures is important, especially if one is embarking on arthroscopic or open debridement of PAI lesions to develop anatomic planes of dissection to preserve as much native structural tissue as possible.

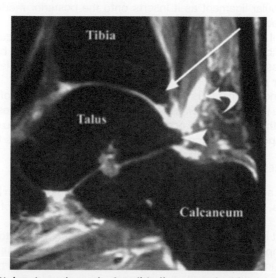

Fig. 6. Sagittal MRI showing a down-sloping tibia (*long arrow*) with a Stieda process (*arrowhead, curved arrow* shows inflammatory changes around FHL).

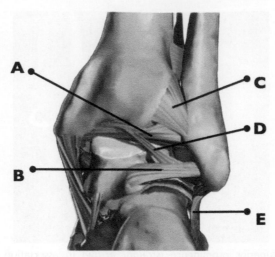

Fig. 7. The posterior ankle ligaments. A, intermalleolar ligament; B, posterior talofibular ligament; C, posterior inferior tibiofibular ligament; D, the tibial slip; E, Calcenofibular ligament.

The PITFL is a thick, stout band running posterior to the interosseous tibiofibular ligament, with which it partly blends. Its medial extent can reach as far as the posterior border of the medial malleolus, and it inserts on the posterior aspect of the fibula. It lies immediately superior to the transverse tibiofibular ligament or intermalleolar ligament, with which it is intimately related, and it too inserts as far medially as the medial malleolus. This ligament can normally form a labrum of the ankle joint by projecting inferiorly to the distal tibia, effectively deepening the tibial articular surface. This ligament is often in contact with the talar articular surface and can potentially split longitudinally or hypertrophy causing labral and synovial impingement.

The tibial slip is a small ligament that is an extension from the upper border of the transverse tibiofibular ligament as it inserts onto the posterior medial tibial plafond and it is connected with the PTFL.

The PTFL is 1 of the 3 lateral ankle joint collateral ligament stabilizers (anterior talofibular, calcaneofibular, posterior talofibular). It is an intracapsular but extrasynovial structure and passes horizontally from the lateral malleolus to the lateral tubercle of the posterior talar process.

The important nonligamentous structure at the posterior aspect of the ankle is the FHL tendon. It lies in a groove between the medial and lateral tubercles of the posterior talar process. At the level of the processes, the tendon enters a fibro-osseous tunnel, which can predispose the tendon to stenotic lesions and contribute to PAI.

CLINICAL FEATURES

Although PAI has several causes, the symptoms on presentation can be similar for the different diseases. The clinician also relies on appropriate imaging of the hindfoot, as discussed later.

In the athlete, it is not unusual for a specific mechanism of injury to be lacking. The patient may complain of pain or discomfort in the ankle when performing certain movements (eg, in soccer, when the player cuts a sudden movement in a certain direction or strikes a ball, or in ballet dancers, when performing relevé positions). This condition is often referred to as an overuse phenomenon. In some series of PAI treatments,[8] half of all athletes presented as an overuse injury, whereas others sustained an acute injury, such as an ankle inversion injury. In classical ballet dancers, probably the commonest form of acute injury to present to the clinician is a forced inversion injury, leading to lateral ankle ligament injury.[9]

If the lateral ligament complex is deficient after a sprain, then during plantarflexion, the talus can rotate anteriorly under the plafond, which could lead to osseous impingement between the tibia and calcaneus.[10] In soccer players, it is often an overuse presentation rather than an acute injury,[11] although injuries such as a PTFL avulsion can lead to PAI.[12] Despite the presence of an acute injury, the onset of symptoms of PAI may be delayed by 3 to 4 weeks.[13] This delay is most likely because in the early inflammatory phase of the injury the athlete is unable to adopt the positions of plantarflexion because of pain, swelling, or hemarthrosis, and as the patient recovers and regains motion the impingement is apparent with either soft tissue hypertrophy or avulsion fragments of bone such as a fracture through an os trigonum synchondrosis.

A thorough history is important, asking about previous injuries sustained or previous treatments, such as therapeutic injections. Many high-level athletes have received injections often to help them finish a season, so there is usually a good correlation between the duration of symptoms in athletes and the number of pain-relieving injections received.[11]

Patients may complain of a feeling of fullness, and swelling may be evident around the back of the ankle (usually laterally rather than medially), unless there is a significant stenosing lesion of the FHL tendon, with resultant tenosynovitis, or a less frequently encountered significant posteromedial impingement lesion as a result of chronic posterior deltoid fiber disruption.[14] Active range of motion may or may not be normal and is not a reliable clinical sign. Ballet dancers may sickle at the ankle to perform relevé positions (ie, they fall into slight inversion to allow for decreased plantarflexion), and this should be looked for in examination. Palpation of the joints can reveal localized areas of inflammation and tenderness, often posterolaterally.

Passive range of motion is a useful examination. Once the area of tenderness is localized, the examiner can recreate exacerbating movements (ie, rapid forced plantarflexion) while palpating the tender area. Pain on examination in combination with crepitus or clicking can be a reliable sign, and a negative result probably excludes the diagnosis, although evidence-based results on its specificity and sensitivity have not been found.

Targeted local anesthesia injection around the clinically defined impingement lesion can be helpful. The forced plantar flexion test can be repeated after injection, and if symptoms are abated, then the diagnosis is clearer and can aid further management.[15]

Examination for FHL tendon problems is important in athletes and dancers. In dancers, repetitive motion of the ankle from plié positions through to relevé positions can irritate the FHL as it travels during extreme ankle dorsiflexion and plantarflexion. to the extent that swelling, crepitus, or a nodule can be felt around the tendon. Examination with resisted plantarflexion of the hallux can exacerbate pain and aid diagnosis. Of particular relevance to the anatomy are those persons with low-lying muscle bellies, where the muscle can become trapped between the tubercles during motion and cause posteromedial ankle pain.[16] Stenosing FHL symptoms can also be commonly seen in athletes who are required to actively flex the hallux during rapid ankle plantarflexion and grounding of the foot (ie, cricket bowlers and javelin throwers).[12] The presence of an os trigonum correlates highly with FHL changes on MRI scans in ballet dancers, with studies[7,17] showing around two-thirds of dancers with significant findings suggestive of FHL tenosynovitis on MRI.

RADIOLOGICAL INVESTIGATIONS
Radiograph

Most clinicians use radiographs as a first-line investigation. Two views are useful. The plain lateral radiograph can detect osseous lesions such as a large os trigonum posteriorly (**Fig. 8**) or a Haglund-type lesion. The posterolateral tubercle of the talus is superimposed on the posteromedial tubercle when looking directly at the lateral projection; Van Dijk[15] recommends rotating the ankle into 25° external rotation to uncover the posterolateral tubercle. The anteroposterior view is generally unhelpful to look specifically for posterior impingement disease.

Computed Tomography Scan

Computed tomography (CT) is an often-overlooked modality of imaging for investigation of ankle impingement. It proves its worth when radiographs fail to diagnose bony impingement lesions even with rotated views and MRI is unable to diagnose subtle, small lesions such as avulsion fragments or irregularities of the surface of the bone, when other features such as bone marrow edema can mask other less obvious bony lesions (**Fig. 9**).[18]

MRI

Accurate use of MRI in interpretation of impingement disease requires a well-informed and experienced radiologist. It is important that your institution has set protocols to ensure that correct sequences are used to diagnose disease. As a minimum, fat-suppressed T2-weighted or proton-density images in the sagittal plane and imaging of the ankle in 3 planes should be requested. The use of contrast-enhanced scans with gadolinium is advised, because this can add subtle detail to differentiate between, for example, synovitis or joint effusion, which has treatment implications.[12]

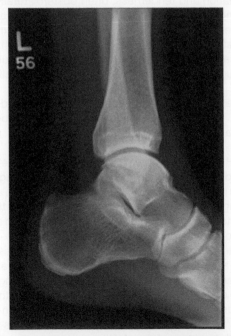

Fig. 8. An os trigonum with a posterosuperior prominence lesion on the calcaneum.

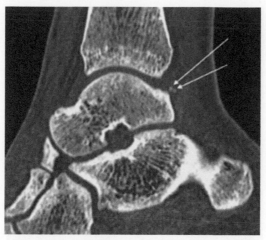

Fig. 9. Sagittal CT scan showing small loose bodies in the posterior aspect of the ankle joint.

Many investigators have detailed the typical findings of PAI on MRI sequences.[7,12,13,17–21] Descriptions of the particular sequences and findings in each is beyond the scope of this article, but there are some important features of PAI to look for.

Osseous

Bone marrow edema can be seen in the posterior talus and the area of the Stieda process or os trigonum (**Fig. 10**). A posterior process fracture of the talus can be seen in some instances (**Fig. 11**). Impingement on dynamic MRI can be seen or static MRI in plantarflexion, with the posterior talus and posterior ligamentous structures impinging between the superior calcaneus and the posterior slope of the tibia (**Fig. 12**).

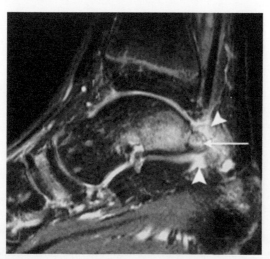

Fig. 10. Talar edema involving the posterior process/os trigonum (*long arrow*), with significant soft tissue edema and inflammation (*arrow heads*).

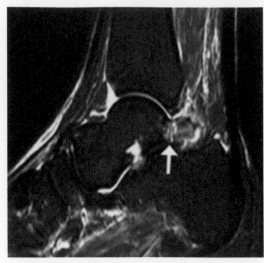

Fig. 11. Posterior process fracture with bony edema.

Soft tissue

Within the ankle, an effusion may be present. The ankle or subtalar capsules can be thickened, more specifically, the posterior ligaments such as the intermalleolar ligament or posterior labrum (**Fig. 13**). Synovitis surrounding the ankle and subtalar joints or the FHL tendon can be marked (**Fig. 14**). On axial MRI, the tenosynovitis can be easily seen around the FHL tendon (**Fig. 15**). On occasion, the muscle belly of the FHL can be low lying, but this is better appreciated during dynamic flexion and extension of the hallux intraoperatively.

Ultrasonography

It seems that with the availability and accuracy of MRI, ultrasonography has a specific and limited role in the investigation and treatment of PAI. Its use is reported for

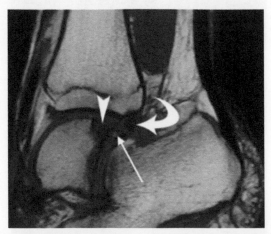

Fig. 12. PAI or the nutcracker phenomenon, with intermalleolar ligament caught in the ankle joint (*curved arrow*) above an os trigonum (*straight arrow*) attached via a synchondrosis (*arrowhead*).

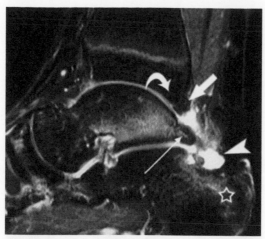

Fig. 13. Thickening of the posterior intermalleolar ligament (*thick straight arrow*), down-sloping tibia (*curved arrow*), Stieda process (*long arrow*), synovitis (*arrowhead*), and calcaneal edema (*star*).

targeted injections with steroid and local anesthesia around the posterior ankle to relieve symptoms.[13,21] It ensures safe injections near neurovascular structures, especially on the medial aspect for FHL symptoms, near the posterior tibial nerve and vessels.

CONSERVATIVE TREATMENT OF PAI

In the athlete, especially the recreational type, a combination of physiotherapy and activity avoidance can produce good results, with marked symptom relief for the

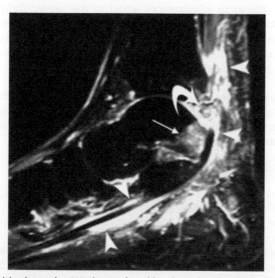

Fig. 14. Tenosynovitis along the FHL (*arrowheads*), talus edema (*small arrow*), and intermalleolar ligament thickening (*curved arrow*).

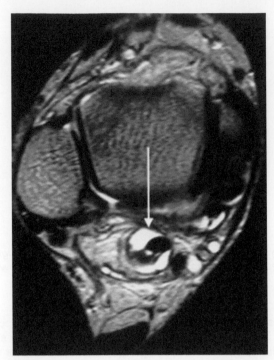

Fig. 15. FHL tenosynovitis, with enhancement around the tendon signifying fluid within the sheath.

treatment of soft tissue or bony impingement lesions.[22] This treatment is largely supported by anecdotal evidence and experience. In the more high-performance and professional athlete, many surgeons use targeted injections to treat the pain symptoms and reduce the local inflammatory effect of the lesion. Before injection, it is important to exclude other diseases that may account for the localized pain, so it is recommended that MRI is performed. Injections can often help athletes finish a season and in some cases prove curative, unless there is a large osseous lesion causing the impingement, in which case repeat injections or resection are almost certainly required.[13,21]

As discussed earlier, the number of injections does correlate with the longevity of the symptoms in the athlete; however, our experience shows that the time to return to function after any surgical intervention (ie, resection or debridement) has no correlation with the number of previous injections received.

OPERATIVE TREATMENT OF PAI
Open Surgery

The open surgical approach, either posteromedial or posterolateral to the ankle and subtalar joint, can be guided by a combination of the patient's symptoms and the lesions seen on imaging. In the senior author's experience of resection of os trigonums in high-level ballet dancers, around two-thirds are through the posteromedial approach. The advantage of the posteromedial approach is the ability to address the FHL tendon and sheath as it passes behind the posterior aspect of the talus directly. Many dancers suffer from concurrent FHL tendinitis with posterior impingement, which can be safely released through this approach.[16] Although the FHL tendon can be released through the posterolateral approach after excision of the impingement lesion (eg, os trigonum), this is not recommended. This technique can have an unacceptably high rate of sural nerve injury (reported to be up to 20%).[23,24] Damage to the posterior tibial nerve is also reported through this posterolateral approach,[25] possibly because of poor visualization of this structure, and it is our opinion that the posteromedial approach should be carefully used if FHL tendon decompression is required. This way the posterior tibial neurovascular bundle can be visualized easily and safely retracted as required, rather than traversing the wound through the posterolateral approach.

Outcomes and return to function after open surgery
In the athlete, open debridement has generally favorable outcomes. Most investigators report around 70% to 80% good or excellent results at latest follow-up.[16,23,25–27] Our experience is that in ballet dancers, open excision (through a posteromedial or posterolateral approach to the hindfoot) of impingement lesions is safe, with neurovascular injuries not encountered. The time to return to full dance in these demanding athletes can be from 9 weeks to 20 weeks. Other investigators report mean return to full sports after open surgery in athletes from 12 to 25 weeks.[16,23,25]

Arthroscopic Surgery

Posterior hindfoot arthroscopy has added another tool to the surgeon's armamentarium for the treatment of this condition.[28] The portal placement and technique with the instruments has been described in a previous issue of this journal.[15] Although this technique has been popularized in recent years,[11,29,30] it can present a technical challenge to the surgeon.

One possible advantage to this approach is an improved view of the posterior ankle structures compared with limited views from open techniques.[12] However, we believe that open procedures when performed through a correctly placed incision can still provide sufficient and safe visual surgical fields. Through the arthroscopic approach, the surgeon can visualize and remove bony lesions either en masse or piecemeal, (ie, os trigonum or Stieda processes). The FHL tendon sheath can also be decompressed to allow free motion of the tendon during movement of the hallux, which can be shown intraoperatively. Other lesions such as ganglions can be seen and removed arthroscopically.

Complications in arthroscopic surgery
The rate of complications seen in published series of posterior ankle arthroscopy is generally low. Wound infection rates are usually 0% to 5%,[31–34] and injury to the sural nerve is reported in a few studies as up to 8%. When injury occurs, it is usually a transient neuropraxia; however, it can be persistent in some cases.[8,30] However, in most studies, the rate of sural nerve injury is 0% to 1%. Some investigators also report patients complaining of numbness, specifically in the posteromedial aspect of the heel.[31,35] Injuries to the posterior tibial nerve have been reported with popularization of arthroscopic techniques, but it is assumed that cases are few and to our knowledge none has been discussed in the literature.

Published data comparing the techniques are lacking. In 1 comparative study, Guo and colleagues[31] reported 1 sural nerve injury in those after open excision and 1 posteromedial calcaneal parasthesia after arthroscopic excision of os trigonums. With care, both techniques should prove safe with minimal to no intraoperative complications.

Outcomes and return to function after arthroscopic surgery
A proposed benefit of arthroscopic excision is the shorter recovery time in athletes and dancers. In the our experience, the return to dance in high-level ballet dancers is variable but can take up to 20 weeks.

In a series of 23 elite soccer players treated arthroscopically for PAI,[11] the return to full play ranged from 29 to 72 days (mean 41 days). The investigators of this study found that the return to function (more specifically, training) was also quicker in those players treated for soft tissue impingement lesions rather than bony impingement lesions. Ten athletes (3 of whom were professional athletes) treated arthroscopically in another study for symptomatic os trigonums returned to sport within 8 weeks.[36] Noguchi and colleagues[8] treated 12 athletes for bony impingement, and the time to return to sport ranged from 3 to 13 weeks (mean 5.9 weeks). These investigators believed that early return to sport was greatly influenced by early mobilization after surgery. Many of the ballet dancers whom we have treated via open methods are immobilized for 1 to 2 weeks to aid wound healing.

The authors of this article have compared open and arthroscopic excision of os trigonums in a retrospective series of high-level ballet dancers. Twenty-two patients (9 male, 13 female) with a mean age of 18 years were treated with open excision, and 13 patients (6 male and 7 female), with a mean age of 20 years, were treated with arthroscopic excision. Neither group experienced any intraoperative or postoperative complications. When the time to return to ballet in the dancers was compared, it was significantly quicker in those treated arthroscopically (mean of 69 days) than after open surgery (mean of 105 days) ($P<.0001$). More of those treated with open excision were younger national ballet school dancers, who are arguably not rehabilitated as aggressively as older, seasoned professional dancers. Differing rehabilitation along with temporary early rigid immobilization, which was used in the open group to aid wound healing, may have contributed to the significant difference in results.

Guo and colleagues' comparative study of 41 athletes from a variety of sports found that the return to dance and playing soccer for those persons after arthroscopic treatment was 6 to 8 weeks in dancers and 4 to 6 weeks in soccer players. In contrast, after open surgery, time to return to dance was 8 to 24 weeks and to soccer, 6 to 12 weeks. The numbers in these sports were small; however, in all these athletes, return to function after arthroscopy was still quicker (6 weeks vs 11.9 weeks, $P<.001$), which echoes the finding of our study.

POSTEROMEDIAL ANKLE IMPINGEMENT

Few reports of this condition are found in the literature. Its importance should not be underestimated, because after successful treatment of anterolateral ligament injuries, patients may continue with deep posteromedial pain in the ankle, which can be debilitating if not recognized. Liu and Mirzayan[37] first described the condition in 1993 in a single case. The mechanism of injury that is often reported is a significant inversion injury. The patient complains of persistent, activity-related pain and swelling posteromedial in the ankle, with localized tenderness on palpation. The posteromedial symptoms at first are usually not apparent compared with the anterolateral symptoms of the likely anterior talofibular ligament injury or even an osteochondral defect; however, as the injury progresses (it may even recur), it is likely that the posteromedial tissues are in a chronic inflammatory state, and as a result, thickening of the ligament and capsule ensues. With repetitive movement, the thickened soft tissue impinges, more specifically, the posterior fibers of the posterior tibiotalar ligament between the posterior aspect of the medial malleolus and the talus. This lesion has been termed a postero-medial impingement (PoMI) lesion.

Mann and Myerson[38] recognized a different type of PoMI lesion, which was secondary to an unossified posteromedial talar tubercle, but still caused similar symptoms. They reported 5 adolescents with a bipartite talus with large posteromedial fragment. Although this is the only series reported, it is worth considering as a cause for posteromedial pain. Other variations in posterior medial talar anatomy can occur, including enlarged posteromedial processes with resulting impingement symptoms (**Fig. 16**).

MRI Findings

When critically examining the posterior tibiotalar ligament on MRI scan, it has lost its normal striation pattern.[39] The posteromedial joint capsule deep to the tibialis posterior tendon can be markedly thickened and in some cases even displace the excursion of the tibialis posterior tendon around the posteromedial aspect of the ankle.[21] Bone bruising in the medial malleolus and corresponding talus indicate abutment lesions impinging on the capsule.[14]

Treatment

In the first report by Liu and Mirzayan,[37] the patient was initially treated conservatively with activity modification. This treatment usually significantly reduces the patient's symptoms, but on resumption of activity, the symptoms quickly recur.[14] Before surgical intervention, it is reasonable to perform a targeted local anesthetic and steroid injection, especially in the athlete wishing to complete a full season. Messiou and colleagues[21] reported that 8 of 9 athletes made a complete return to sport within 3 weeks after an injection, with only 1 requiring surgery, for what was an enlarged posteromedial process of the talus.

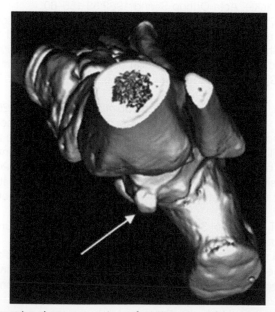

Fig. 16. Three-dimensional reconstruction of a CT scan, with an enlarged posteromedial talar tubercle in a soccer player.

Surgical intervention is described both through posteromedial direct open excision[14] and via anterior ankle arthroscopy in the manner described by Foetisch and Ferkel.[40]

SUMMARY

PAI can dramatically reduce athletes' performance. The history can be of either a specific traumatic event, or in many cases, an overuse-type phenomenon. Focused clinical examination can pinpoint the location of the lesion. CT can be used in the investigation strategy and diagnosis of small bony impingement lesions/fragments, especially when MRI or plain radiographs fail to show major soft tissue or bony disease. Ultrasound-guided injections are useful to help locate the symptomatic lesions and also reduce the level of symptoms sufficiently to enable a player to finish a season. Injections may occasionally cure soft tissue impingement lesions; however, in bony impingement lesions, symptoms likely recur, necessitating surgical excision for resolution of symptoms. Posterior arthroscopic surgical excision of true posterior impingement lesions is recommended, with significantly quicker return to sport expected; however, open excision remains an option.

ACKNOWLEDGMENTS

The authors would like to thank Kate Jones for her assistance in preparing some of the figures.

REFERENCES

1. Rasmussen O, Tovborg-Jensen I. Mobility of the ankle joint: recording of rotatory movements in the talocrural joint in vitro with and without the lateral collateral ligaments of the ankle. Acta Orthop Scand 1982;53:155–60.
2. Hamilton WG, Hamilton LH, Marshall P, et al. A profile of the musculoskeletal characteristics of elite professional ballet dancers. Am J Sports Med 1992;20:267–73.
3. Russell JA, Shave RM, Kruse DW, et al. Ankle and foot contributions to extreme plantar- and dorsiflexion in female ballet dancers. Foot Ankle Int 2011;32:183–8.
4. Lawson JP. Symptomatic radiographic variants in extremities. Radiology 1985; 157:625–31.
5. McDougall A. The os trigonum. J Bone Joint Surg Br 1955;37:257–65.
6. van Dijk CN, van Sterkenburg MN, Wiegerinck JI, et al. Terminology for Achilles tendon related disorders. Knee Surg Sports Traumatol Arthrosc 2011;19:835–41.
7. Peace KA, Hillier JC, Hulme A, et al. MRI features of posterior ankle impingement syndrome in ballet dancers: a review of 25 cases. Clin Radiol 2004;59:1025–33.
8. Noguchi H, Ishii Y, Takeda M, et al. Arthroscopic excision of posterior ankle bony impingement for early return to the field: short-term results. Foot Ankle Int 2010; 31:398–403.
9. Hardaker WT, Margello S, Goldner JL. Foot and ankle injuries in theatrical dancers. Foot Ankle 1985;6:59–69.
10. Hamilton WG. Posterior ankle pain in dancers. Clin Sports Med 2008;27:263–77.
11. Calder JD, Sexton SA, Pearce CJ. Return to training and playing after posterior ankle arthroscopy for posterior impingement in elite professional soccer. Am J Sports Med 2010;38:120–4.
12. Lee JC, Calder JD, Healy JC. Posterior impingement syndromes of the ankle. Semin Musculoskelet Radiol 2008;12:154–69.

13. Robinson P, Bollen SR. Posterior ankle impingement in professional soccer players: effectiveness of sonographically guided therapy. AJR Am J Roentgenol 2006;187:W53–8.
14. Paterson RS, Brown JN. The posteromedial impingement lesion of the ankle. A series of six cases. Am J Sports Med 2001;29:550–7.
15. van Dijk CN. Anterior and posterior ankle impingement. Foot Ankle Clin 2006;11: 663–83.
16. Hamilton WG, Geppert MJ, Thompson FM. Pain in the posterior aspect of the ankle in dancers. Differential diagnosis and operative treatment. J Bone Joint Surg Am 1996;78:1491–500.
17. Bureau NJ, Cardinal E, Hobden R, et al. Posterior ankle impingement syndrome: MR imaging findings in seven patients. Radiology 2000;215:497–503.
18. Masciocchi C, Catalucci A, Barile A. Ankle impingement syndromes. Eur J Radiol 1998;27(Suppl 1):S70–3.
19. Wakeley CJ, Johnson DP, Watt I. The value of MR imaging in the diagnosis of the os trigonum syndrome. Skeletal Radiol 1996;25:133–6.
20. Donovan A, Rosenberg ZS. MRI of ankle and lateral hindfoot impingement syndromes. AJR Am J Roentgenol 2010;195:595–604.
21. Messiou C, Robinson P, O'Connor PJ, et al. Subacute posteromedial impingement of the ankle in athletes: MR imaging evaluation and ultrasound guided therapy. Skeletal Radiol 2006;35:88–94.
22. Albisetti W, Ometti M, Pascale V, et al. Clinical evaluation and treatment of posterior impingement in dancers. Am J Phys Med Rehabil 2009;88:349–54.
23. Abramowitz Y, Wollstein R, Barzilay Y, et al. Outcome of resection of a symptomatic os trigonum. J Bone Joint Surg Am 2003;85:1051–7.
24. Veazey BL, Heckman JD, Galindo MJ, et al. Excision of ununited fractures of the posterior process of the talus: a treatment for chronic posterior ankle pain. Foot Ankle 1992;13:453–7.
25. Marotta JJ, Micheli LJ. Os trigonum impingement in dancers. Am J Sports Med 1992;20:533–6.
26. Leutloff D, Perka C. Posterior ankle impingement syndrome in dancers–a short-term follow-up after operative treatment. Foot Ankle Surg 2002;8:33–9.
27. Spicer DD, Howse AJ. Posterior block of the ankle: the results of surgical treatment in dancers. Foot Ankle Surg 1999;5:187–90.
28. van Dijk CN, Scholten PE, Krips R. A 2-portal endoscopic approach for diagnosis and treatment of posterior ankle pathology. Arthroscopy 2000;16:871–6.
29. Willits K, Sonneveld H, Amendola A, et al. Outcome of posterior ankle arthroscopy for hindfoot impingement. Arthroscopy 2008;24:196–202.
30. Galla M, Lobenhoffer P. Technique and results of arthroscopic treatment of posterior ankle impingement. Foot Ankle Surg 2011;17:79–84.
31. Guo QW, Hu YL, Jiao C, et al. Open versus endoscopic excision of a symptomatic os trigonum: a comparative study of 41 cases. Arthroscopy 2010;26: 384–90.
32. Allegra F, Maffulli N. Double posteromedial portals for posterior ankle arthroscopy in supine position. Clin Orthop Relat Res 2010;468:996–1001.
33. Nickisch F, Barg A, Saltzman CL, et al. Postoperative complications of posterior ankle and hindfoot arthroscopy. J Bone Joint Surg Am 2012;94:439–46.
34. Horibe S, Kita K, Natsu-ume T, et al. A novel technique of arthroscopic excision of a symptomatic os trigonum. Arthroscopy 2008;24:121.e1–4.
35. Scholten PE, Sierevelt IN, Van Dijk CN. Hindfoot endoscopy for posterior ankle impingement. J Bone Joint Surg Am 2008;90:2665–72.

36. Jerosch J, Fadel M. Endoscopic resection of a symptomatic os trigonum. Knee Surg Sports Traumatol Arthrosc 2006;14:1188–93.
37. Liu SH, Mirzayan R. Posteromedial ankle impingement. Arthroscopy 1993;9: 709–11.
38. Mann HA, Myerson MS. Treatment of posterior ankle pain by excision of a bipartite talar fragment. J Bone Joint Surg Br 2010;92:954–7.
39. Koulouris G, Connell D, Schneider T, et al. Posterior tibiotalar ligament injury resulting in posteromedial impingement. Foot Ankle Int 2003;24:575–83.
40. Foetisch CA, Ferkel RD. Deltoid ligament injuries: anatomy, diagnosis, and treatment. Sports Med Arthrosc Rev 2001;8:326.

Acute Achilles Tendon Rupture in Athletes

Umile Giuseppe Longo, MD, MSc, PhD[a,b,*], Stefano Petrillo, MD[a,b],
Nicola Maffulli, MD, MS, PhD, FRCS(Orth)[c], Vincenzo Denaro, MD[a,b]

KEYWORDS

- Achilles tendon rupture • Operative repair of achilles • Athlete

KEY POINTS

- Athletes require operative repair of the Achilles tendon following acute rupture.
- The choice of open versus percutaneous techniques continues to be debated.
- Early rehabilitation should be instigated: early movement and weight bearing leads to improved tendon healing.

INTRODUCTION

The Achilles tendon (AT) is the strongest and largest tendon in the human body, and is also the most frequently ruptured.[1,2] AT rupture is more common in men, with a male/female ratio of between 1.7:1 and 30:1. However, ATs in men present higher stiffness and maximum rupture force than in women, and also have a larger cross-sectional area.[3] Moreover, younger tendons present significantly higher tensile rupture stress despite having lower stiffness.[4] The incidence of AT ruptures has largely increased in the last decade,[5,6] and they usually occur in sedentary, white-collar individuals who play sport occasionally, mostly in the third or fourth decade of life.[7] Therefore, most AT ruptures (44%–83%) occur during sport activities, and biochemical and biomechanical changes related to aging may play a significant role in the pathogenesis of the injury.[8] Subcutaneous tears are more common in the AT compared with any other tendon in human body. Several microscopic interruptions in the tendinous substance occur during normal activities, whereas fibers remodel and new collagen is continuously formed.[9,10] A tendon usually loses its wavy configuration when stretched more than 2%. When the tendon is stretched by more than 3% to 4% of its normal length, it starts to disrupt, and, when stretched more than 8%, macroscopic rupture occurs.[11]

[a] Department of Orthopaedic and Trauma Surgery, Campus Bio-Medico University, Via Alvaro del Portillo, 200, Trigoria, Rome 00128, Italy; [b] Centro Integrato di Ricerca (CIR), Campus Bio-Medico University, Via Alvaro del Portillo, 21, Rome 00128, Italy; [c] Centre for Sports and Exercise Medicine, Barts and The London School of Medicine and Dentistry, Mile End Hospital, 275 Bancroft Road, London E1 4DG, England
* Corresponding author.
E-mail address: g.longo@unicampus.it

Foot Ankle Clin N Am 18 (2013) 319–338
http://dx.doi.org/10.1016/j.fcl.2013.02.009
1083-7515/13/$ – see front matter © 2013 Elsevier Inc. All rights reserved.
foot.theclinics.com

ANATOMY AND HISTOLOGY

The AT consists of the tendinous portions of the gastrocnemius and soleus muscles. Moreover, the plantaris muscle is present in 93% (752 of 810) of lower extremities, located medially to the AT and distinct from it.[12] The medial and lateral heads of the gastrocnemius originate from the femoral condyles and their contribution to the AT commences as a wide aponeurosis at the lower ends of these muscular bellies.[12] The soleus muscle originates from the tibia and fibula, and its tendinous contribution to the Achilles tendon is shorter and thicker.[12] The calcaneal insertion is composed of a specialized layer of hyaline cartilage and an area of bone not covered by periosteum. A retrocalcanear bursa is located between the AT and the calcaneus, whereas a subcutaneous bursa is located between the tendon and the skin.[13] The cellular population of the tendon is composed of tenocytes and tenoblasts for 90% to 95%, whereas collagen and elastin proteins account for 70% and 2% of the dry weight of a tendon, respectively, and form most of the extracellular matrix (ECM).[14] Type I collagen is the most common, and it accounts for 95% of tendon collagen,[15] whereas tenocytes from ruptured ATs produce more type III collagen than tenocytes from normal ATs,[16] which is less resistant and elastic to tensile force. The ground substance of ECM surrounding the collagen and the tenocytes is composed of glycoproteins, glycosaminoglycans, and proteoglycans.[17] Glycosaminoglycans decrease with aging, whereas collagen increases, and acute exercise increases the formation of type I collagen in the peritendinous tissue.[18,19] The tendon is formed by well-organized fascicles surrounded by endotenon. These fascicles are enveloped by a layer of connective tissue, the epitenon, in direct contact with the endotenon.[20–22] The epitenon, in turn, is surrounded by the paratenon with a thin layer of fluid in between to allow tendon movement with reduced friction.[23] Type I and type III collagen fibrils, an inner lining of synovial cells, and few elastin fibrils compose the paratenon, which is in contact with the fascia cruris covering the posterior aspect of the tendon.[24] In addition, the paratenon has 2 layers: a superficial layer called the peritenon, which is connected with the underlying layer via the mesotenon; and a deeper layer, surrounding and in direct contact with the epitenon.[24] The sensory supply of the AT derives from the nerves of the attaching muscles and cutaneous nerves, in particular the sural nerve.[25] Moreover, the AT blood supply is guaranteed proximally by the musculotendinous junction, along its length by the surrounding connective tissue, and distally by the bone-tendon junction.[26] The site of AT rupture is usually 2 to 6 cm proximal to the tendon insertion. The poor vascularity in the main body of the AT may play an important role in the pathogenesis of the rupture.[27] Furthermore, the blood flow is higher in women compared with controls, and decreases with aging.[28] Exercise increases the blood flow 4-fold in the AT 5 cm proximal to the insertion, whereas it increases only 2.5-fold 2 cm proximal to the insertion.[29]

CAUSES AND PATHOLOGY

Several hypotheses have been developed to clarify the causes of AT rupture, but there is no agreement in the literature,[30] and the events leading to an AT rupture are still unclear.[31–33] Numerous factors such as gastrocnemius-soleus dysfunction, a suboptimally conditioned musculotendinous unit, age, gender, changes in training pattern, poor technique, previous injuries, footwear,[34,35] poor tendon vascularity, and degeneration[36,37] are frequently attributed to AT ruptures. In addition, various pathologic conditions, such as infectious diseases, neurologic conditions,[38] hyperthyroidism, renal insufficiency, arteriosclerosis,[39] inflammatory and autoimmune conditions, hyperuricemia, genetically determined collagen abnormalities,[40] and high serum lipid concentration,[41,42] can be associated with AT ruptures.

Two main theories are proposed for the cause of AT ruptures: the degenerative theory and the mechanical theory. The degenerative theory states that the chronic degeneration of the tendon leads to a rupture without excessive loads being applied. The degeneration of the tendon tissue can be caused by numerous factors such as chronic overloading or microtrauma, physiologic alterations in the tendon, and pharmacologic treatments.

Degenerative Theory

The molecular events leading to a rupture of the AT are still unclear.[31–33] Arner and colleagues[43] were the first to observe degenerative changes in all of their patients with AT rupture. They hypothesized that these changes were already present before the rupture, although their data were obtained more than 2 days after the rupture. Davidsson and Salo[44] found degenerative changes in 2 patients with AT rupture operated on the day of injury, and they also concluded that the degenerative changes were already present before the rupture.[45] Similar findings were obtained in our own series. In all of the ATs operated on within 24 hours after the injury, we detected marked degenerative changes and collagen disruption.[46,47] Moreover, several investigators observed degenerative alterations in the intratendinous substance of the AT in various patients with a spontaneous rupture, in all sites studied, and most of these abnormalities had no known cause.[47] Several investigators have hypothesized that alterations in blood flow with subsequent hypoxia and impaired metabolism were important factors for the development of the degenerative changes of the AT. Kannus and Jozsa[48] evaluated patients with spontaneous AT ruptures using biopsy specimens, harvested at the time of repair. They noted that only a small proportion of the patients presented symptoms before the rupture, suggesting that degenerative changes are common in the tendons of people who are older than 35 years, and that these changes can be associated with spontaneous rupture.[48] These observations were confirmed by another study of ours. In the 176 AT ruptures that we treated from January 1990 to December 1996, only 9 (5%) patients had had previous symptoms.[49] We also showed that tenocytes from ruptured and tendinopathic tendons produced type III collagen, which alters the physiologic tissue architecture, making the tissue less resistant to high loads and tensile forces.[49] Furthermore, Jozsa and colleagues[50] observed that fibronectin, which is normally located in basement membranes, was present on the torn surfaces of ruptured ATs. Fibronectin is present in a soluble form in plasma, and binds more readily to denatured collagen than to normal collagen, indicating pre-existing collagen denaturation.[51]

Mechanical Theory

The AT can be damaged when frequent and repetitive microtrauma occur, without leaving enough time to the tendon for repair,[52,53] even in healthy tendons with no degeneration.[54] Numerous movements occurring in many sports, and not just those that require rapid push-off, may be responsible for these occurrences. A healthy AT usually ruptures after a violent muscular strain in the presence of an incomplete synergism of agonist muscle contractions, inefficient action of the plantaris muscle acting as a tensor of the AT, and a discrepancy in the thickness quotient between muscle and tendon.[54] Inglis and Sculco[34] suggested that uncoordinated muscle contractions could cause a rupture of an otherwise normal tendon, and athletes who have a long period of inactivity and return to training too early seem to present a greater risk of a rupture caused by this mechanism. Sporting activity plays a major role in the development of problems with the AT, especially when training session are wrongly performed.[35] Moreover, the risk of rupture of the AT is greatly increased during inversion or eversion movements of the subtalar joint when they are associated with the application of oblique stress. AT injury may also result from structural or dynamic disturbances in normal lower leg mechanics such as functional overpronation, gastrocnemius/soleus insufficiency, overtraining, and repeated microtrauma produced by the eccentric loading of fatigued muscle.[55] In conclusion, complete rupture of the AT can be considered as the consequence of multiple microtrauma and microruptures that lead to failure of the tendon after reaching a critical point.[56]

Drug-related Tendon Rupture

Drugs such as anabolic steroids and fluoroquinolones cause dysplasia of collagen fibrils, which decreases tendon tensile strength and increases the risk of AT rupture.

Normal and healthy tendons are not usually damaged by intratendinous injection of steroids,[57] whereas systemic and local corticosteroid administration have been widely implicated in tendon rupture.[58,59] Nevertheless, numerous studies have shown that the intratendinous or peritendinous injection of corticosteroids into an injured tendon may precipitate a rupture.[57,60] In addition, the analgesic properties of corticosteroids may mask or delay the onset of the symptoms related to damage to the tendon,[61] inducing individuals to maintain their high activity levels even when the tendon is damaged. Corticosteroids also interfere with the healing of tendons, resulting in collagen necrosis. The consequent restoration of tendon strength is attributable to the formation of a cellular amorphous mass of collagen, and, for these reasons, vigorous physical activity should be avoided for at least 2 weeks following injection of corticosteroids close to a tendon.[62]

The administration of the fluoroquinolone (4-quinolone) antibiotics or ciprofloxacin has been associated with tendon rupture. Pefloxacin, ofloxacin, levofloxacin, norfloxacin, and ciprofloxacin are the fluoroquinolones most frequently associated with tendon disorders. A variety of laboratory evidence for the direct deleterious effects of fluoroquinolones on tenocytes has been produced.[63] In a study conducted on 100 patients taking fluoroquinolones, several tendon disorders were observed, including 31 ruptures.[64] However, numerous patients in this study also received corticosteroids. In addition, in an animal study the administration of fluoroquinolone was associated with disruption of the ECM of cartilage, depletion of collagen, and necrosis of chondrocytes, suggesting that these abnormalities in animals might also occur in humans.[65]

Mechanism of Rupture

According to Arner and Lindholm,[66] the mechanisms of AT rupture can be classified into 3 main categories:

1. Fifty-three percent of ruptures occur during weight bearing with the forefoot pushing off and the knee in extension. Sprint starts and jumping sports more often require these movements and this explains the prevalence of left AT rupture in right-handed people.
2. Seventeen percent of ruptures occur following sudden unexpected dorsiflexion of the ankle, such as slipping into a hole, or falling downstairs.
3. In 10% of patients, the tendon was ruptured because of violent dorsiflexion of a plantarflexed foot, such as may occur after falling from a height. In the rest of their patients, they could not identify the mechanism of injury.

PRESENTATION AND DIAGNOSIS

The diagnosis of AT ruptures should start with a careful assessment of the history followed by physical examination.[38,67] Nevertheless, 20% to 25% of AT ruptures are not diagnosed by the first examining doctor,[11,68,69] whereas the clinical diagnosis is immediate in case of acute ruptures of the AT.

Patients with ruptured ATs usually report a history of pain in the affected leg and the feeling that, at the time of injury, they had been kicked in the posterior aspect of the lower leg. Moreover, the inability to bear weight and weakness or stiffness of the affected ankle are common. However, a small number of patients may be still able to use the flexor hallucis longus, flexor digitorum longus, tibialis posterior, and peroneal tendons to plantarflex the affected ankle.

On clinical examination, diffuse edema and bruising are usually present, and, unless the swelling is severe, a palpable gap may be felt along the course of the tendon, most frequently 2 to 6 cm proximal to the insertion of the tendon.[70] Inspection and palpation should be followed by other tests to confirm the diagnosis, such as the Simmonds and Matles test and the O'Brien and Copeland tests.

The Simmonds or Thompson calf squeeze test is performed with the patient prone on the examination couch and the ankles off the couch, and the examiner squeezes the fleshy part of the calf. This procedure causes the overlying of the AT, producing plantar flexion of the ankle if the tendon is intact.[71] The clinical findings on the affected leg following this test should be compared with the opposite leg to exclude any false positive that may occur in the presence of an intact plantaris tendon.[72]

The Matles test is performed with the patient prone on the examination couch. Patients are asked to flex their knees to 90°, and, if the foot on the affected side falls into neutral or dorsiflexion position, an AT rupture is diagnosed.[73]

The O'Brien test consists of the insertion of a hypodermic 25-gauge needle through the skin of the calf, medial to the midline and 10 cm proximal to the superior border of the calcaneus, within the substance of the tendon. The ankle is then alternately plantarflexed and dorsiflexed and if, on dorsiflexion, the needle point moves distally, the tendon is presumed to be intact in the portion distal to the needle. If, on dorsiflexion, the needle point moves proximally or remains still, there is presumed to be a loss of continuity between the needle and the site of tendon insertion.[69]

The Copeland test is performed by asking the patient to lie prone with the knee flexed to 90° and a sphygmomanometer cuff positioned around the bulk of the calf of the affected leg. The cuff is then inflated to 100 mm Hg with the foot in plantarflexion. The foot is then dorsiflexed. If the pressure increases to approximately 140 mm Hg, the musculotendinous unit is presumed to be intact. The opposite leg should be used to exclude a false-positive response or for comparison purposes.[74]

IMAGING EVALUATION

Real-time high-resolution ultrasonography and magnetic resonance imaging are more sensitive and less invasive imaging evaluations than soft tissue radiography or xeroradiography. However, ultrasonography is generally considered the primary imaging method for the diagnosis of AT ruptures.[75,76]

Lateral radiographs of the ankle can be performed to diagnose an AT rupture. The loss of normal configuration of the Kager triangle, the space between the anterior aspect of the AT, the posterior aspect of the tibia, and the superior aspect of the calcaneum, is pathognomonic of AT rupture. Arner and colleagues[43] found that deformation of the contours of the distal segment of the tendon resulting from loss of tone were the radiographic changes most likely to be associated with AT rupture. The Toygar sign[77] involves measuring the angle of the posterior skin surface curve seen on plain radiographs, because the ends of the tendon are displaced anteriorly following a complete tear. The posterior aspect of the Kager triangle then approaches the anterior aspect, and the triangle decreases or disappears. An angle of 130° to 150° indicates AT rupture.

Ultrasonography of the AT is considered the primary imaging method to diagnose a rupture, although it is operator dependent.[75,76] The possibility of performing a dynamic and panoramic evaluation of the AT by means of linear ultrasonography is influenced by the type of transducer used and the angle of the ultrasound beam with respect to the tendon.[78] Moreover, ultrasonography can be used to evaluate the tendon structure after any kind of operative repair. Despite their short focusing distance, high-frequency probes of 7.5 to 10 MHz provide the best resolution.[79] To avoid artifacts during the ultrasonography evaluation of the AT, the probe should be managed by expert examiners and held at right angles to the tendon. Linear array transducers are therefore more suitable than sector-type transducers, which produce excess obliquity of the ultrasound beam at the edges. It may also be necessary to use a synthetic gel spacer or standoff pad, increasing the definition of the surface echoes and allowing a suitable support.[80,81] The normal ultrasonography appearance of the AT is a ribbonlike hypoechogenic image, contained within 2 hyperechogenic bands. Tendon fascicles appear as alternate hypoechogenic and hyperechogenic bands that are more compact when the tendon is strained and more separated when the tendon is relaxed.[80] The presence of an acoustic vacuum with thick, irregular edges is typical in AT rupture.[80]

The normal aspect of the AT in magnetic resonance imaging is hypointense on all pulse sequences. The Kager triangle, which appears hyperintense because of the presence of fat, is well delineated by the AT. Sagittal-plane and axial-plane T1-weighted and T2-weighted images are usually used to evaluate suspected AT ruptures, especially in cases of increase in intratendinous signal intensity (**Fig. 1**). In T1-weighted images, the AT rupture appear as disruption of the signal within the tendon, whereas in T2-weighted images the rupture is seen as a generalized increase in signal intensity. Moreover, in T2-weighted images, the edema and hemorrhage at the site of rupture are seen as an area of high signal intensity.

MANAGEMENT OF ACUTE AT RUPTURE

The management of acutely ruptured AT can be broadly classified into operative and nonoperative[82] and usually depends on the preference of the surgeon and the patient. The surgical management consists of open or percutaneous repair, whereas the conservative management consists of immobilization or functional bracing. More evidence is available for the use of percutaneous techniques than for open surgery,[83,84] and also for the use of early mobilization.[85–87]

Surgical treatment has been the method of choice in the last 2 decades, especially in athletes and young people and in cases of delayed ruptures, whereas conservative, nonoperative management can be used in nonathletes.[88] Open operative management of acute AT ruptures significantly reduces the risk of rerupture compared with nonoperative treatment, but is associated with a significantly higher risk of wound healing problems,[89] which can be reduced by performing surgery percutaneously.[82,83]

The objective of the management of AT rupture is to minimize the morbidity of the injury, optimize rapid return to full function, and prevent complications. The complications can be rated as major or minor from their impact on daily life activities, and can be divided into 3 categories: (1) wound complications, (2) general complications; and

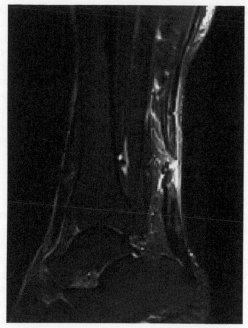

Fig. 1. Magnetic resonance imaging showing a complete AT rupture, identifying disruptions of the signal within the tendon.

(3) rerupture. Deep venous thrombosis, pulmonary embolism, and rerupture are the most severe complications and may affect patients regardless of treatment.[89]

NONOPERATIVE MANAGEMENT

Conservative management and percutaneous repair can be considered viable alternatives to open surgery, which is the most risky and costly of the 3 options.[82] The choice of the type of management should take into account the age, occupation, and level of sporting activity of each patient.

Pels Leusden was the first to propose nonoperative management for AT rupture, in the early 1900s.[90] Immobilization in a below-knee plaster cast in gravity equinus position for 4 weeks followed by a more neutral position for a further 4 weeks is considered the most common nonoperative protocol of management of AT rupture.[91–96] Other investigators maintained the gravity equinus position for 2 weeks, followed by a more neutral position for a further 2 weeks. After this period, a below-knee plaster cast with the foot plantigrade is applied for a further 2 weeks, allowing weight bearing for the last 2 weeks of this management regime. After 1 to 3 weeks of immobilization, braces, splints, or shoes with limitation of dorsiflexion and increased heel height have been used for functional rehabilitation.[97–100] The reports on early functional treatment suggest good functional outcome and low rerupture rates.[101]

In elderly patients, more than 70 years of age, who present chronic AT rupture, physiotherapy alone can be used. These patients usually complain of weakness in plantar flexion and of a strange gait, but they often adapt well to their disability.

Following immobilization, a profound alteration of muscle morphology and physiology occur.[102] Aside from the gastrocnemius muscle, which is a biarticular muscle able to move when a short leg cast is used, the soleus muscle is particularly susceptible to immobilization. Because of the presence of a high proportion of type I muscle fibers in the human soleus, it is particularly susceptible to atrophy if immobilized.[103] Problems caused by immobilization may also occur after open operative management, but not to the same extent as with nonoperative management. The calf circumference greatly decreases after nonoperative management compared with operative management.[104] Moreover, following operative management, no significant difference of calf circumference is seen compared with the uninjured contralateral tendon.[104] However, patients with open operative repairs spend less time in plaster, and are more often are serious athletes who comply well with postoperative management (**Fig. 2**).

Immobilization

Plaster cast immobilization, usually for a period of 6 to 10 weeks, is most commonly used,[105] and the clinical outcome is comparable with operative management.[94,106] Although function following nonoperative repair is generally good, the high incidence of rerupture is considered unacceptable. Lea and Smith[94] reported a rerupture rate of 13% in 55 spontaneously ruptured ATs, managed with below-the-knee cast immobilization for 8 weeks with the foot in gravity equinus, followed by a 2.5-cm heel lift for a further 4 weeks after cast removal. Persson and Wredmark[96] reported a 35% rate of rerupture in 20 patients managed nonoperatively. Moreover, at the final followup, 16 patients had no complaints, the remaining 4 had only minor problems, and 7 patients, not necessarily those whose tendon had reruptured, were not satisfied with the result. Using functional bracing, McComis and colleagues[98] nonoperatively treated 15 patients who had sustained a rupture of the AT. Good functional results were achieved in all patients, suggesting that, in selected cases, functional bracing may be a viable alternative to the use of plaster cast or operative intervention for the management of acute ruptures of the AT.

SURGICAL MANAGEMENT
Percutaneous Repair

In 1977, Ma and Griffith[107] were the first to propose percutaneous repair for the management of AT ruptures, to find a compromise between open surgical and nonsurgical management. After producing 6 small stab incisions across the medial and lateral borders of the tendon, they passed a suture through the tendon using

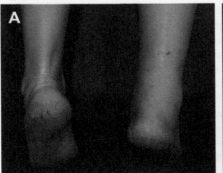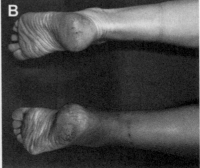

Fig. 2. (*A*, *B*) Ruptures of the AT and results after conservative treatment with cast.

these incisions. There were no reruptures, but 2 minor, noninfectious skin complications occurred. Similar results were obtained by FitzGibbons and colleagues[108] concerning rerupture rate; no skin infections occurred, but there was a case of sural nerve injury. In our previous center in Aberdeen, United Kingdom, Rowley and Scotland[109] described 24 patients with rupture of the AT, 14 treated by casting in equinus position alone, and 10 treated by percutaneous repair. One patient with percutaneous repair suffered entrapment of the sural nerve, but no other complications were encountered. Moreover, patients in the sutured group reached earlier normal plantar flexion strength and normal activity than the group treated by cast alone. In contrast, numerous investigators report a lower success rate with percutaneous repair. Klein and colleagues[110] reported sural nerve entrapment in 13% of 38 patients. Hockenbury and Johns[111] performed an in vitro study using a transverse tenotomy of the ATs extracted from 10 fresh frozen below-the-knee cadaver specimens who received percutaneous AT repair or open AT repair. The specimens were divided into 2 groups of 5 specimens each, 1 receiving open Achilles repair using a Bunnell suture technique, the other undergoing percutaneous repair according to the Ma and Griffith[107] technique. The ATs undergoing open repair were able to resist almost twice the amount of ankle dorsiflexion than those undergoing percutaneous repair before a 10-mm gap in the repaired tendon appeared (27.6° vs 14.4°, $P<.05$). In addition, entrapment of the sural nerve occurred in 3 of 5 specimens undergoing percutaneous repair and the tendon stumps were malaligned in 4 of 5 specimens. Since this study, percutaneous repair of AT ruptures has been associated with approximately 50% of the initial strength guaranteed by open repair, and places the sural nerve at higher risk for injury. Furthermore, in most studies, , percutaneous repair is associated with a higher rerupture rate compared with open operative repair.[112] Also, high rates of transfixion of the sural nerve have been reported,[109,111] with persistent paresthesias and the necessity of formal exploration to remove the suture and free the nerve.[110]

In 2005, Webb and Bannister[113] described a new percutaneous repair technique, performed under local anesthesia using 3 midline transverse 2.5-cm incisions over the posterior aspect of the AT. No reruptures or sural nerve injuries occurred at a median interval of 35 months after the injury. We later modified this technique using stronger absorbable sutures and a Kessler suture,[114] and Carmont and Maffulli[115] presented a modification of the previously described technique. This modification, which uses 3 transverse incisions, minimizes the chance of sural nerve injury, allowing an even less invasive approach to the tendon that permits the accurate apposition of the tendon ends. Ismail and colleagues[116] compared the mechanical properties of the Achillon mini-incision technique with the long-established Kessler method, concluding that the strength of the repair was related to tendon diameter and that there were no differences between the two techniques. We prefer the Carmont and Maffulli[115] technique compared with the Achillon repair: the first procedure is cheaper, and creates a stronger repair, because it allows the use of a greater number of suture strands (8) for the repair of the AT. However, we conducted a biomechanical study comparing the primary stability of Achillon repair and our modified percutaneous repair[115] on 18 (9 matched pairs) frozen ovine ATs, concluding that the Achillonlike configuration and the modified percutaneous repair of ruptured AT provided similar biomechanical performance.[117]

Despite the high risk of skin wound problems, several advantages are associated with open surgical repair of AT ruptures, such as correct alignment of the torn tendon, excellent functional results with less chance of rerupture, superior strength, and early active mobilization.

Percutaneous Repair Preferred by the Authors

The patient's position is prone (**Fig. 3**).[115] A 20-mL solution of 1% lignocaine is used to infiltrate the areas 4 to 6 cm proximal and distal to the palpable tendon defect and the skin over the lesion. Ten milliliters of Chirocaine 0.5% are infiltrated deep to the tendon defect. A calf tourniquet is applied to exsanguinate the limb. The skin preparation and draping are performed in a standard fashion. A size 11 blade is used to perform a 1-cm transverse incision over the defect and 4 longitudinal stab incisions are made on the lateral and medial aspects of the AT, 4 and 6 cm proximally to the palpable defect. In addition, 2 longitudinal incisions on either side of the tendon aspect are made proximally to the calcaneal insertion of the tendon. The tendon is then mobilized from the subcutaneous tissue by means of forceps. A 9-cm Mayo needle (BL059N, #B00 round-point spring eye, B. Braun, Aesculap, Tuttlingen, Germany) is threaded with 2 double loops of number 1 Maxon (Tyco Healthcare, Norwalk, CT), and this is passed transversely between the proximal stab incisions through the bulk of the tendon. The

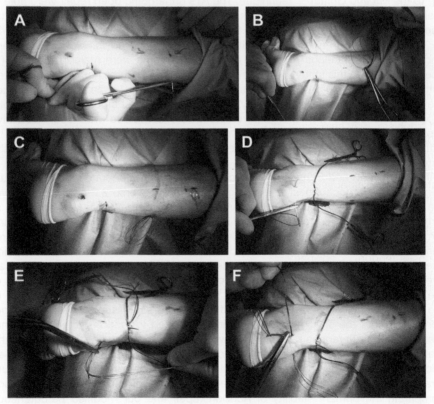

Fig. 3. (*A*) A 9-cm Mayo needle (BL059N, #B00 round-point spring eye, B Braun, Aesculap, Tuttlingen, Germany) is threaded with 2 double loops of number 1 Maxon (Tyco Healthcare, Norwalk, CT), and is passed transversely between the proximal stab incisions through the bulk of the tendon. (*B, C*) Each of the ends is then passed distally from just proximal to the transverse Maxon passage through the bulk of the tendon to pass out of the diagonally opposing stab incision. (*D*) Another double loop of Maxon is passed between the distal stab incisions through the tendon and (*E, F*) in turn through the tendon and out of the transverse incision starting distal to the transverse passage.

bulk of the tendon is superficial. The loose ends are held with a clip. In turn, each of the ends is then passed distally from just proximal to the transverse Maxon passage through the bulk of the tendon to pass out of the diagonally opposing stab incision. A subsequent diagonal pass is then made to the transverse incision over the ruptured tendon. Clips are used to hold both ends of the Maxon, preventing entanglement. To test the security of this suture, both ends of the Maxon are pulled distally. In addition, the distal stab incision through the tendon is used to pass another double loop of Maxon, and in turn through the tendon and out of the transverse incision starting distal to the transverse passage. The ankle is held in full plantar flexion, and in turn opposing ends of the Maxon thread are tied together with a double throw knot, and then 3 further throws, before being buried using forceps. To maintain the tension of the suture, another clip is used to hold the first throw of the lateral side. The transverse incision is closed with a subcuticular Biosyn suture 3.0 (Tyco Healthcare) and Steri-strips (3M Health Care, St Paul, MN) are used to close the stab incisions. At the end, a Mepore dressing (Molnlycke Health Care, Gothenburg, Sweden) is applied, and a bivalved removable scotch cast with Velcro straps is used to position the foot in full plantar flexion.

Open Surgical Repair

In recent years, open surgical repair was considered the gold standard for the management of AT ruptures in young, fit individuals (**Fig. 4**). Moreover, the numerous advances in surgical techniques, such as in postoperative rehabilitation protocols, have encouraged many surgeons to favor direct tendon repair.[39] In addition, the excellent results of surgical repair concerning rerupture rates and tendon strength, such as calf trophism, may help many athletes to return to preinjury physical activities.

Different operative techniques can be performed to repair ruptured ATs, ranging from simple end-to-end suturing by Bunnell or Kessler sutures, to more complex repairs using fascial reinforcement or tendon grafts,[118] artificial tendon implants, materials such as absorbable polymer–carbon fiber composites,[119] xenograft ECM scaffolds,[120,121] Marlex mesh, and collagen tendon prostheses.[122] Primary augmentation of the repair with the plantaris tendon,[123] a single central or 2 (1 medial, 1 lateral) gastrocnemius fascial turndown flaps,[124] the peroneus brevis tendon,[125] the gracil tendon,[126] the bone-patellar tendon,[127] the bone-quadriceps tendon,[128] the semitendinosus tendon,[129] and the free hamstring tendon transfer[130] was also performed. However, there is no evidence that, in acute AT ruptures, this is better than a nonaugmented end-to-end repair.[131] Platelet–rich plasma (PRP) has also been used alone for the management of chronic AT tendinopathy,[132] or in association with open repair in case of acute AT ruptures (**Fig. 5**).[133] Randomized control trials that evaluated the role

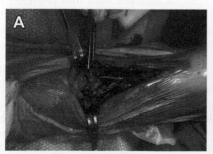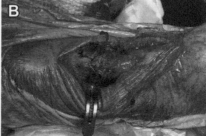

Fig. 4. (A, B) Open surgical repair of an acute AT rupture.

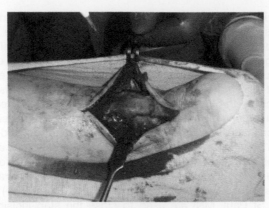

Fig. 5. Application of PRP after open surgical repair of an acute AT rupture.

of PRP in acutely ruptured AT or in chronic AT tendinopathy concluded that PRP is not useful for the management of these disorders.[132,133] In our opinion, the use of augmentation should be preferred only when dealing with delayed repairs, chronic tears, and in the management of reruptures.[125,126,134–139]

POSTOPERATIVE MANAGEMENT

Patients can be discharged 2 days after or the same date as the operation, if any complication occurs. An orthopedic physiotherapist should instruct the patient to use crutches. Patients are allowed to bear weight on the operated leg as tolerated. In addition, is important to tell the patient to keep the affected leg elevated for as long as possible to prevent swelling. Patients are followed on an outpatient basis at 2-week intervals, and the cast is removed 6 weeks after the operation.[85,86] In case of application of a cast with the ankle in equinus, after this period it is changed, putting the ankle in gradually increasing dorsiflexion, until plantigrade, after 2 and 4 weeks. The cast is then removed 6 weeks after the operation.[140] After the 6-week immobilization period, patients should weight bear partially, and gradual stretching and strengthening exercises are allowed. Full weight bearing is not advised before 8 to 10 weeks after surgery. During the period in the cast, gentle isometric contractions of the gastro-soleus complex must be started, especially after weight bearing has become comfortable. After removal of the cast, patients should start to mobilize the ankle and, after 2 weeks, cycling and swimming are permitted, also continuing the active ankle mobilization exercises. Patients usually return to their normal sports activity 4 months after the surgery.[85–87]

In athletes, postoperative management must be different from that provided for nonathletic patients. The ankle must be immobilized in equinus position with an anterior below-knee plaster-of-Paris slab. Patients are usually discharged on the same day or the day after the operation. They are allowed to toe-touch weight bear on the operated limb as tolerated. They are also advised to keep the operated leg elevated for as long as possible, to reduce postoperative swelling. After 48 to 72 hours, when the postoperative swelling should be significantly reduced, patients are seen in the plaster room to change the plaster-of-Paris slab with an anterior below-knee synthetic slab with the ankle in gravity equinus. The slab is kept in place by an elastic bandage, which allows plantar flexion of the ankle, whereas dorsiflexion is limited by the foot piece of the slab. Patients must use crunches and are allowed to weight bear as tolerated. The slab is changed at the second postoperative week so that the ankle can dorsiflex to neutral, and dorsiflexion is limited until the sixth week, when the slab is removed. When high-level, well-motivated athletes are compliant, they can usually return to some training 6 to 8 weeks after the removal of the anterior slab. The anterior slab can be substituted with a hinged orthosis, which is more expensive than a simple synthetic cast but can be reused. Moreover, free ankle motion after repair of AT provided by a patellar tendon bearing plaster cast with a protecting frame under the foot, allowing weight bearing immediately after surgery, is also safe and associated with satisfactory clinical results.[141] The preinjury level of sporting activity is usually reached 4 months after surgery.[85–87]

OUTCOME EVALUATION

The variables usually studied after AT rupture are complications to treatment, calf muscle strength, patient satisfaction, endurance, tendon configuration, impact of AT rupture on absence from work, and impact on sports participation. Overall, outcome measurements using 100-point scoring systems have been used.[4,98,142,143] The major limitation to their common use has been that the scores include dynamometry testing, which are not widely available in routine clinical practice.

The AT Total Rupture Score[144] can be a good solution to resolve this problem. It is a patient-reported instrument for measuring outcome after treatment of total AT rupture. It is a self-administered instrument with high clinical usefulness, and it has been suggested for measuring the outcome, related to symptoms and physical activity, after treatment in patients with total AT rupture.

SUMMARY

In recent decades, the incidence of AT rupture has increased, whereas the evidence for best management is still debated, and several options are still challenging. In elderly or a few selected patients, conservative management and early mobilization achieves excellent results but the associated rerupture rate is not acceptable in young individuals. Open surgery is frequently associated with higher risk of superficial skin breakdown and wound problems, which can be prevented by performing percutaneous repair. Percutaneous repair, performed under local anesthesia and followed by early functional rehabilitation, is becoming increasingly common, and may be considered in selected patients. However, several percutaneous techniques are proposed by different investigators, and there is a lack of appropriate trials that show which of these is the best. More randomized controlled trials are awaited to clarify the issues and disputes discussed in this article.

REFERENCES

1. Ames PR, Longo UG, Denaro V, et al. Achilles tendon problems: not just an orthopaedic issue. Disabil Rehabil 2008;30(20–22):1646–50.
2. Maffulli N, Waterston SW, Squair J, et al. Changing incidence of Achilles tendon rupture in Scotland: a 15-year study. Clin J Sport Med 1999;9:157–60.
3. Longo UG, Rittweger J, Garau G, et al. No influence of age, gender, weight, height, and impact profile in Achilles tendinopathy in masters track and field athletes. Am J Sports Med 2009;37:1400–5.
4. Thermann H, Frerichs O, Biewener A, et al. Biomechanical studies of human Achilles tendon rupture. Unfallchirurg 1995;98:570–5 [in German].
5. Jarvinen TA, Kannus P, Maffulli N, et al. Achilles tendon disorders: etiology and epidemiology. Foot Ankle Clin 2005;10:255–66.

6. Moller A, Astron M, Westlin N. Increasing incidence of Achilles tendon rupture. Acta Orthop Scand 1996;67:479–81.
7. Schepsis AA, Jones H, Haas AL. Achilles tendon disorders in athletes. Am J Sports Med 2002;30:287–305.
8. Landvater SJ, Renstrom PA. Complete Achilles tendon ruptures. Clin Sports Med 1992;11:741–58.
9. Longo UG, Ronga M, Maffulli N. Achilles tendinopathy. Sports Med Arthrosc 2009;17:112–26.
10. Longo UG, Ronga M, Maffulli N. Acute ruptures of the Achilles tendon. Sports Med Arthrosc 2009;17:127–38.
11. Maffulli N. Rupture of the Achilles tendon. J Bone Joint Surg Am 1999;81: 1019–36.
12. Cummins EJ, Anson BJ, Carr BW, et al. The structure of the calcaneal tendon (of Achilles) in relation to orthopedic surgery. Surg Gynecol Obstet 1946;83: 107–16.
13. Rufai A, Ralphs JR, Benjamin M. Structure and histopathology of the insertional region of the human Achilles tendon. J Orthop Res 1995;13:585–93.
14. Robins SP. Functional properties of collagen and elastin. Baillieres Clin Rheumatol 1988;2:1–36.
15. Kader D, Saxena A, Movin T, et al. Achilles tendinopathy: some aspects of basic science and clinical management. Br J Sports Med 2002;36:239–49.
16. Maffulli N, Ewen SW, Waterston SW, et al. Tenocytes from ruptured and tendinopathic Achilles tendons produce greater quantities of type III collagen than tenocytes from normal Achilles tendons. An in vitro model of human tendon healing. Am J Sports Med 2000;28:499–505.
17. Kannus P, Jozsa L, Jarvinnen M. Basic science of tendons. In: Garrett WJ, Speer K, Kirkendall DT, editors. Principles and practice of orthopaedic sports medicine. Philadelphia: Lippincott Williams & Wilkins; 2000. p. 21–37.
18. Vailas AC, Pedrini VA, Pedrini-Mille A, et al. Patellar tendon matrix changes associated with aging and voluntary exercise. J Appl Physiol 1985;58: 1572–6.
19. Langberg H, Skovgaard D, Petersen LJ, et al. Type I collagen synthesis and degradation in peritendinous tissue after exercise determined by microdialysis in humans. J Physiol 1999;521(Pt 1):299–306.
20. Denaro V, Ruzzini L, Longo UG, et al. Effect of dihydrotestosterone on cultured human tenocytes from intact supraspinatus tendon. Knee Surg Sports Traumatol Arthrosc 2010;18:971–6.
21. Knobloch K, Schreibmueller L, Longo UG, et al. Eccentric exercises for the management of tendinopathy of the main body of the Achilles tendon with or without an AirHeel brace. A randomized controlled trial. B: Effects of compliance. Disabil Rehabil 2008;30:1692–6.
22. Knobloch K, Schreibmueller L, Longo UG, et al. Eccentric exercises for the management of tendinopathy of the main body of the Achilles tendon with or without the AirHeel brace. A randomized controlled trial. A: effects on pain and microcirculation. Disabil Rehabil 2008;30:1685–91.
23. Longo UG, Oliva F, Olivia F, et al. Oxygen species and overuse tendinopathy in athletes. Disabil Rehabil 2008;30:1563–71.
24. Kvist H, Kvist M. The operative treatment of chronic calcaneal paratenonitis. J Bone Joint Surg Br 1980;62:353–7.
25. Stilwell DL Jr. The innervation of tendons and aponeuroses. Am J Anat 1957; 100:289–317.

26. Carr AJ, Norris SH. The blood supply of the calcaneal tendon. J Bone Joint Surg Br 1989;71:100–1.
27. Astrom M, Westlin N. Blood flow in chronic Achilles tendinopathy. Clin Orthop Relat Res 1994;166–72.
28. Schmidt-Rohlfing B, Graf J, Schneider U, et al. The blood supply of the Achilles tendon. Int Orthop 1992;16:29–31.
29. Langberg H, Bulow J, Kjaer M. Blood flow in the peritendinous space of the human Achilles tendon during exercise. Acta Physiol Scand 1998;163:149–53.
30. Maffulli N, Irwin AS, Kenward MG, et al. Achilles tendon rupture and sciatica: a possible correlation. Br J Sports Med 1998;32:174–7.
31. Karousou E, Ronga M, Vigetti D, et al. Collagens, proteoglycans, MMP-2, MMP-9 and TIMPs in human Achilles tendon rupture. Clin Orthop Relat Res 2008;466:1577–82.
32. Campani R, Bottinelli O, Genovese E, et al. The role of echotomography in sports traumatology of the lower extremity. Radiol Med 1990;79:151–62 [in Italian].
33. Carden DG, Noble J, Chalmers J, et al. Rupture of the calcaneal tendon. The early and late management. J Bone Joint Surg Br 1987;69:416–20.
34. Inglis AE, Sculco TP. Surgical repair of ruptures of the tendo Achillis. Clin Orthop Relat Res 1981;160–9.
35. Clain MR, Baxter DE. Achilles tendinitis. Foot Ankle 1992;13:482–7.
36. Maffulli N. Achilles tendon rupture. Br J Sports Med 1995;29:279–80.
37. Williams JG. Achilles tendon lesions in sport. Sports Med 1993;16:216–20.
38. Maffulli N. Clinical tests in sports medicine: more on Achilles tendon. Br J Sports Med 1996;30:250.
39. Myerson MS. Achilles tendon ruptures. Instr Course Lect 1999;48:219–30.
40. Dent CM, Graham GP. Osteogenesis imperfecta and Achilles tendon rupture. Injury 1991;22:239–40.
41. Mathiak G, Wening JV, Mathiak M, et al. Serum cholesterol is elevated in patients with Achilles tendon ruptures. Arch Orthop Trauma Surg 1999;119:280–4.
42. Ozgurtas T, Yildiz C, Serdar M, et al. Is high concentration of serum lipids a risk factor for Achilles tendon rupture? Clin Chim Acta 2003;331:25–8.
43. Arner O, Lindholm A, Orell SR. Histologic changes in subcutaneous rupture of the Achilles tendon; a study of 74 cases. Acta Chir Scand 1959;116:484–90.
44. Davidsson L, Salo M. Pathogenesis of subcutaneous tendon ruptures. Acta Chir Scand 1969;135:209–12.
45. Jozsa L, Kannus P, Balint JB, et al. Three-dimensional ultrastructure of human tendons. Acta Anat (Basel) 1991;142:306–12.
46. Jarvinen M, Jozsa L, Kannus P, et al. Histopathological findings in chronic tendon disorders. Scand J Med Sci Sports 1997;7:86–95.
47. Jozsa L, Kannus P. Histopathological findings in spontaneous tendon ruptures. Scand J Med Sci Sports 1997;7:113–8.
48. Kannus P, Jozsa L. Histopathological changes preceding spontaneous rupture of a tendon. A controlled study of 891 patients. J Bone Joint Surg Am 1991;73:1507–25.
49. Waterston SW, Maffulli N, Ewen SW. Subcutaneous rupture of the Achilles tendon: basic science and some aspects of clinical practice. Br J Sports Med 1997;31:285–98.
50. Jozsa L, Lehto M, Kannus P, et al. Fibronectin and laminin in Achilles tendon. Acta Orthop Scand 1989;60:469–71.

51. Lehto M, Jozsa L, Kvist M, et al. Fibronectin in the ruptured human Achilles tendon and its paratenon. An immunoperoxidase study. Ann Chir Gynaecol 1990;79:72–7.
52. Hayes T, McClelland D, Maffulli N. Metasynchronous bilateral Achilles tendon rupture. Bull Hosp Jt Dis 2003;61:140–4.
53. Selvanetti A, Cipolla M, Puddu G. Overuse tendon injuries: basic science and classification. Oper Tech Sports Med 1997;5:110–7.
54. Barfred T. Experimental rupture of the Achilles tendon. Comparison of various types of experimental rupture in rats. Acta Orthop Scand 1971;42:528–43.
55. Clement DB, Taunton JE, Smart GW. Achilles tendinitis and peritendinitis: etiology and treatment. Am J Sports Med 1984;12:179–84.
56. Knorzer E, Folkhard W, Geercken W, et al. New aspects of the etiology of tendon rupture. An analysis of time-resolved dynamic-mechanical measurements using synchrotron radiation. Arch Orthop Trauma Surg 1986;105:113–20.
57. Matthews LS, Sonstegard DA, Phelps DB. A biomechanical study of rabbit patellar tendon: effects of steroid injection. J Sports Med 1974;2:349–57.
58. Newnham DM, Douglas JG, Legge JS, et al. Achilles tendon rupture: an underrated complication of corticosteroid treatment. Thorax 1991;46:853–4.
59. Dickey W, Patterson V. Bilateral Achilles tendon rupture simulating peripheral neuropathy: unusual complication of steroid therapy. J R Soc Med 1987;80: 386–7.
60. Unverferth LJ, Olix ML. The effect of local steroid injections on tendon. J Sports Med 1973;1:31–7.
61. DiStefano VJ, Nixon JE. Ruptures of the Achilles tendon. J Sports Med 1973;1: 34–7.
62. Kennedy JC, Willis RB. The effects of local steroid injections on tendons: a biomechanical and microscopic correlative study. Am J Sports Med 1976;4:11–21.
63. Bernard-Beaubois K, Hecquet C, Hayem G, et al. In vitro study of cytotoxicity of quinolones on rabbit tenocytes. Cell Biol Toxicol 1998;14:283–92.
64. Royer RJ, Pierfitte C, Netter P. Features of tendon disorders with fluoroquinolones. Therapie 1994;49:75–6.
65. Szarfman A, Chen M, Blum MD. More on fluoroquinolone antibiotics and tendon rupture. N Engl J Med 1995;332:193.
66. Arner O, Lindholm A. Subcutaneous rupture of the Achilles tendon; a study of 92 cases. Acta Chir Scand Suppl 1959;116:1–51.
67. Maffulli N. Current concepts in the management of subcutaneous tears of the Achilles tendon. Bull Hosp Jt Dis 1998;57:152–8.
68. Maffulli N. The clinical diagnosis of subcutaneous tear of the Achilles tendon. A prospective study in 174 patients. Am J Sports Med 1998;26:266–70.
69. O'Brien T. The needle test for complete rupture of the Achilles tendon. J Bone Joint Surg Am 1984;66:1099–101.
70. DiStefano VJ, Nixon JE. Achilles tendon rupture: pathogenesis, diagnosis, and treatment by a modified pullout wire technique. J Trauma 1972;12:671–7.
71. Scott BW, al Chalabi A. How the Simmonds-Thompson test works. J Bone Joint Surg Br 1992;74:314–5.
72. Simmonds FA. The diagnosis of the ruptured Achilles tendon. Practitioner 1957; 179:56–8.
73. Matles AL. Rupture of the tendo Achilles. Another diagnostic sign. Bull Hosp Joint Dis 1975;36:48–51.
74. Copeland SA. Rupture of the Achilles tendon: a new clinical test. Ann R Coll Surg Engl 1990;72:270–1.

75. Bleakney RR, Tallon C, Wong JK, et al. Long-term ultrasonographic features of the Achilles tendon after rupture. Clin J Sport Med 2002;12:273–8.
76. Rolf C, Movin T. Etiology, histopathology, and outcome of surgery in achillodynia. Foot Ankle Int 1997;18:565–9.
77. Toygar O. Subkutane ruptur der Achillesschne (diagnostik und behandlungser-gebnisse). Helv Chir Acta 1947;14:209–31.
78. Maffulli N, Dymond NP, Capasso G. Ultrasonographic findings in subcutaneous rupture of Achilles tendon. J Sports Med Phys Fitness 1989;29:365–8.
79. Fornage BD. Achilles tendon: US examination. Radiology 1986;159:759–64.
80. Barbolini G, Monetti G, Montorsi A, et al. Results with high-definition sonography in the evaluation of Achilles tendon conditions. It J Sports Traumatology 1988; 10:225–34.
81. Maffulli N, Dymond NP, Regine R. Surgical repair of ruptured Achilles tendon in sportsmen and sedentary patients: a longitudinal ultrasound assessment. Int J Sports Med 1990;11:78–84.
82. Ebinesan AD, Sarai BS, Walley GD, et al. Conservative, open or percutaneous repair for acute rupture of the Achilles tendon. Disabil Rehabil 2008; 30(20–22):1721–5.
83. Khan RJ, Fick D, Keogh A, et al. Treatment of acute Achilles tendon ruptures. A meta-analysis of randomized, controlled trials. J Bone Joint Surg Am 2005;87: 2202–10.
84. Longo UG, Ramamurthy C, Denaro V, et al. Minimally invasive stripping for chronic Achilles tendinopathy. Disabil Rehabil 2008;30(20–22):1709–13.
85. Maffulli N, Tallon C, Wong J, et al. Early weightbearing and ankle mobilization after open repair of acute midsubstance tears of the Achilles tendon. Am J Sports Med 2003;31:692–700.
86. Maffulli N, Tallon C, Wong J, et al. No adverse effect of early weight bearing following open repair of acute tears of the Achilles tendon. J Sports Med Phys Fitness 2003;43:367–79.
87. Maffulli N. Immediate weight-bearing is not detrimental to operatively or conser-vatively managed rupture of the Achilles tendon. Aust J Physiother 2006;52:225.
88. Farizon F, Pages A, Azoulai JJ, et al. Surgical treatment of ruptures of the Achilles tendon. Apropos of 42 cases treated by Bosworth's technique. Rev Chir Orthop Reparatrice Appar Mot 1997;83:65–9 [in French].
89. Saxena A, Maffulli N, Nguyen A, et al. Wound complications from surgeries per-taining to the Achilles tendon: an analysis of 219 surgeries. J Am Podiatr Med Assoc 2008;98:95–101.
90. Stein SR, Luekens CA Jr. Closed treatment of Achilles tendon ruptures. Orthop Clin North Am 1976;7:241–6.
91. Edna TH. Non-operative treatment of Achilles tendon ruptures. Acta Orthop Scand 1980;51:991–3.
92. Gillies H, Chalmers J. The management of fresh ruptures of the tendo Achillis. J Bone Joint Surg Am 1970;52:337–43.
93. Jacobs D, Martens M, Van Audekercke R, et al. Comparison of conservative and operative treatment of Achilles tendon rupture. Am J Sports Med 1978;6:107–11.
94. Lea RB, Smith L. Non-surgical treatment of tendo Achillis rupture. J Bone Joint Surg Am 1972;54:1398–407.
95. Lildholdt T, Munch-Jorgensen T. Conservative treatment to Achilles tendon rupture. A follow-up study of 14 cases. Acta Orthop Scand 1976;47:454–8.
96. Persson A, Wredmark T. The treatment of total ruptures of the Achilles tendon by plaster immobilisation. Int Orthop 1979;3:149–52.

97. Saleh M, Marshall PD, Senior R, et al. The Sheffield splint for controlled early mobilisation after rupture of the calcaneal tendon. A prospective, randomised comparison with plaster treatment. J Bone Joint Surg Br 1992;74:206–9.

98. McComis GP, Nawoczenski DA, DeHaven KE. Functional bracing for rupture of the Achilles tendon. Clinical results and analysis of ground-reaction forces and temporal data. J Bone Joint Surg Am 1997;79:1799–808.

99. Eames MH, Eames NW, McCarthy KR, et al. An audit of the combined non-operative and orthotic management of ruptured tendo Achillis. Injury 1997;28:289–92.

100. Thermann H, Hufner T, Tscherne H. Achilles tendon rupture. Orthopade 2000;29:235–50 [in German].

101. Wong J, Barrass V, Maffulli N. Quantitative review of operative and nonoperative management of Achilles tendon ruptures. Am J Sports Med 2002;30:565–75.

102. Qin L, Appell HJ, Chan KM, et al. Electrical stimulation prevents immobilization atrophy in skeletal muscle of rabbits. Arch Phys Med Rehabil 1997;78:512–7.

103. Vrbova G. Changes in the motor reflexes produced by tenotomy. J Physiol 1963;166:241–50.

104. Haggmark T, Liedberg H, Eriksson E, et al. Calf muscle atrophy and muscle function after non-operative vs operative treatment of Achilles tendon ruptures. Orthopedics 1986;9:160–4.

105. Fierro NL, Sallis RE. Achilles tendon rupture. Is casting enough? Postgrad Med 1995;98:145–52.

106. Stein SR, Luekens CA. Methods and rationale for closed treatment of Achilles tendon ruptures. Am J Sports Med 1976;4:162–9.

107. Ma GW, Griffith TG. Percutaneous repair of acute closed ruptured Achilles tendon: a new technique. Clin Orthop Relat Res 1977;247–55.

108. FitzGibbons RE, Hefferon J, Hill J. Percutaneous Achilles tendon repair. Am J Sports Med 1993;21:724–7.

109. Rowley DI, Scotland TR. Rupture of the Achilles tendon treated by a simple operative procedure. Injury 1982;14:252–4.

110. Klein W, Lang DM, Saleh M. The use of the Ma-Griffith technique for percutaneous repair of fresh ruptured tendo Achillis. Chir Organi Mov 1991;76:223–8.

111. Hockenbury RT, Johns JC. A biomechanical in vitro comparison of open versus percutaneous repair of tendon Achilles. Foot Ankle 1990;11:67–72.

112. Bradley JP, Tibone JE. Percutaneous and open surgical repairs of Achilles tendon ruptures. A comparative study. Am J Sports Med 1990;18:188–95.

113. Webb JM, Bannister GC. Percutaneous repair of the ruptured tendo Achillis. J Bone Joint Surg Br 1999;81:877–80.

114. McClelland D, Maffulli N. Percutaneous repair of ruptured Achilles tendon. J R Coll Surg Edinb 2002;47:613–8.

115. Carmont MR, Maffulli N. Modified percutaneous repair of ruptured Achilles tendon. Knee Surg Sports Traumatol Arthrosc 2008;16:199–203.

116. Ismail M, Karim A, Shulman R, et al. The Achillon Achilles tendon repair: is it strong enough? Foot Ankle Int 2008;29:808–13.

117. Longo UG, Forriol F, Campi S, et al. A biomechanical comparison of the primary stability of two minimally invasive techniques for repair of ruptured Achilles tendon. Knee Surg Sports Traumatol Arthrosc 2012;20:1392–7.

118. Soma CA, Mandelbaum BR. Repair of acute Achilles tendon ruptures. Orthop Clin North Am 1995;26:239–47.

119. Parsons JR, Rosario A, Weiss AB, et al. Achilles tendon repair with an absorbable polymer-carbon fiber composite. Foot Ankle 1984;5:49–53.

120. Wisbeck JM, Parks BG, Schon LC. Xenograft scaffold full-wrap reinforcement of Krackow Achilles tendon repair. Orthopedics 2012;35:e331–4.
121. Magnussen RA, Glisson RR, Moorman CT. Augmentation of Achilles tendon repair with extracellular matrix xenograft: a biomechanical analysis. Am J Sports Med 2011;39:1522–7.
122. Kato YP, Dunn MG, Zawadsky JP, et al. Regeneration of Achilles tendon with a collagen tendon prosthesis. Results of a one-year implantation study. J Bone Joint Surg Am 1991;73:561–74.
123. Quigley TB, Scheller AD. Surgical repair of the ruptured Achilles tendon. Analysis of 40 patients treated by the same surgeon. Am J Sports Med 1980;8: 244–50.
124. Ponnapula P, Aaranson RR. Reconstruction of Achilles tendon rupture with combined V-Y plasty and gastrocnemius-soleus fascia turndown graft. J Foot Ankle Surg 2010;49:310–5.
125. Maffulli N, Spiezia F, Pintore E, et al. Peroneus brevis tendon transfer for reconstruction of chronic tears of the Achilles tendon: a long-term follow-up study. J Bone Joint Surg Am 2012;94:901–5.
126. Maffulli N, Spiezia F, Testa V, et al. Free gracilis tendon graft for reconstruction of chronic tears of the Achilles tendon. J Bone Joint Surg Am 2012;94: 906–10.
127. Miyamoto W, Takao M, Matsushita T. Reconstructive surgery using autologous bone-patellar tendon graft for insertional Achilles tendinopathy. Knee Surg Sports Traumatol Arthrosc 2012;20:1863–7.
128. Philippot R, Wegrzyn J, Grosclaude S, et al. Repair of insertional Achilles tendinosis with a bone-quadriceps tendon graft. Foot Ankle Int 2010;31:802–6.
129. Sarzaeem MM, Lemraski MM, Safdari F. Chronic Achilles tendon rupture reconstruction using a free semitendinosus tendon graft transfer. Knee Surg Sports Traumatol Arthrosc 2012;20:1386–91.
130. Maffulli N, Longo UG, Spiezia F, et al. Free hamstrings tendon transfer and interference screw fixation for less invasive reconstruction of chronic avulsions of the Achilles tendon. Knee Surg Sports Traumatol Arthrosc 2010;18:269–73.
131. Jessing P, Hansen E. Surgical treatment of 102 tendo Achillis ruptures– suture or tenontoplasty? Acta Chir Scand 1975;141:370–7.
132. de Vos RJ, Weir A, van Schie HT, et al. Platelet-rich plasma injection for chronic Achilles tendinopathy: a randomized controlled trial. JAMA 2010;303:144–9.
133. Schepull T, Kvist J, Norrman H, et al. Autologous platelets have no effect on the healing of human Achilles tendon ruptures: a randomized single-blind study. Am J Sports Med 2011;39:38–47.
134. Maffulli N, Ajis A, Longo UG, et al. Chronic rupture of tendo Achillis. Foot Ankle Clin 2007;12:583–96, vi.
135. Maffulli N, Longo UG, Gougoulias N, et al. Ipsilateral free semitendinosus tendon graft transfer for reconstruction of chronic tears of the Achilles tendon. BMC Musculoskelet Disord 2008;9:100.
136. Maffulli N, Leadbetter WB. Free gracilis tendon graft in neglected tears of the Achilles tendon. Clin J Sport Med 2005;15:56–61.
137. Carmont MR, Maffulli N. Less invasive Achilles tendon reconstruction. BMC Musculoskelet Disord 2007;8:100.
138. Maffulli N, Ajis A. Management of chronic ruptures of the Achilles tendon. J Bone Joint Surg Am 2008;90:1348–60.
139. Pintore E, Barra V, Pintore R, et al. Peroneus brevis tendon transfer in neglected tears of the Achilles tendon. J Trauma 2001;50:71–8.

140. Coutts A, MacGregor A, Gibson J, et al. Clinical and functional results of open operative repair for Achilles tendon rupture in a non-specialist surgical unit. J R Coll Surg Edinb 2002;47:753–62.
141. Solveborn SA, Moberg A. Immediate free ankle motion after surgical repair of acute Achilles tendon ruptures. Am J Sports Med 1994;22:607–10.
142. Leppilahti J, Forsman K, Puranen J, et al. Outcome and prognostic factors of Achilles rupture repair using a new scoring method. Clin Orthop Relat Res 1998;152–61.
143. Moller M, Karlsson J, Lind K, et al. Tissue expansion for repair of severely complicated Achilles tendon ruptures. Knee Surg Sports Traumatol Arthrosc 2001;9:228–32.
144. Nilsson-Helander K, Thomee R, Gravare-Silbernagel K, et al. The Achilles tendon total rupture score (ATRS): development and validation. Am J Sports Med 2007;35:421–6.

Stress Fractures of the Tibia and Medial Malleolus

Benjamin C. Caesar, MD, MBBS, FRCS Ed (Orth), FRCS, Dip SEM[a],
Graham A. McCollum, FCS Orth(SA), MMED(UCT)[a],
Robin Elliot, MA, FRCS(Tr&Orth)[b], Andy Williams, FRCS(Orth), FFSEM(UK)[a],
James D.F. Calder, TD, MD, FRCS(Tr&Orth), FFSEM(UK)[a,c,*]

KEYWORDS

• Stress fracture • Tibia • Medial malleolus • Athlete

KEY POINTS

• Stress fractures of the medial malleolus are not common, but can occur in athletes manifesting as activity-related pain around the medial side of the ankle with or without ankle swelling and stiffness.

• Only about 30% of fractures are visible on radiographs but bone scan and magnetic resonance imaging have almost 100% sensitivity in diagnosing the fracture.

• Conservative management of tibial stress fractures is frequently successful, but high-risk fractures such as those of the anterior tibial diaphyseal cortex and the medial malleolus may require early operative intervention.

• Intramedullary nail fixation appears effective in tibial diaphyseal fractures and compression screw fixation for medial malleolar fractures, but controversy surrounds whether the stress fracture site should be drilled/debrided and the use of adjuvant therapy such as therpaeutic ultrasound and shockwave therapy.

INTRODUCTION

Stress fracture and stress reactions are a continuum of conditions. Stress reaction precedes stress fracture and is a radiological term to reflect the magnetic resonance imaging (MRI) appearance of periosteal reaction and bone marrow edema. They are fatigue-failure injuries of bone caused by overuse, resulting in a mechanical failure of bone following an accumulation of microdamage secondary to repetitive strain episodes.

Stress fractures in the general population are rare; the reported incidence in a large epidemiologic study from Edinburgh reported an incidence of 0.5% for spontaneous or stress fractures in all bones over the course of a year in a well-defined population.[1] However, stress fractures are considerably more common in the athletic population;

[a] Department of Orthopaedic Surgery, Chelsea & Westminister Hospital, 369 Fulham Road, London SW10 9NH, UK; [b] Hampshire Hospitals NHS Trust, Aldermaston Road, Basingstoke, Hampshire RG24 9AL, UK; [c] Fortius Clinic, 17 Fitzhardinge Street, London W1H 6EQ, UK
* Corresponding author. Fortius Clinic, 17 Fitzhardinge Street, London W1H 6EQ, UK
E-mail address: james.calder@imperial.ac.uk

Foot Ankle Clin N Am 18 (2013) 339–355
http://dx.doi.org/10.1016/j.fcl.2013.02.010
1083-7515/13/$ – see front matter © 2013 Elsevier Inc. All rights reserved.

the figures from Matheson and colleagues'[2] 1987 article suggest that most of these injuries are sustained in the tibia (49.1%), followed by the tarsals (25.3%), metatarsals (8.8%), femur (7.2%), fibula (6.6%), pelvis (1.6%), sesamoids (0.9%), and spine (0.6%). The difficulties in accurately ascertaining the incidence figures for these injuries is summarized well in the article by Snyder and colleagues,[3] where they highlight the need for large prospective studies to delineate the risks of stress fracture by sport, age, and gender. Although the need for such research is present, it may not be practical for such studies to be reported because of the relatively small number of cases and mobility of the population affected.

The incidence of stress fractures in military recruits is subject to much investigation and numerous articles have been published on the subject with varying incidences reported, depending on the training environment under study. Armstrong and coworkers reported that approximately 5% of all military recruits (US Navy) incur stress fracture injuries during intense physical training, predominately in the lower extremity.[4] In a prospective study of 295 male Israeli military recruits by Milgrom et al, they found a 31% incidence of stress fractures. Eighty percent of the fractures were in the tibial or femoral shaft, whereas only 8% occurred in the tarsus and metatarsus. Sixty-nine percent of the femoral stress fractures were asymptomatic, but only 8% of those were in the tibia.[5]

Stress fractures have been classified into high and low risk by multiple authors.[6–8] In the low-risk category are posteromedial tibial fractures, along with fractures of the femoral diaphysis, ribs, ulna shaft, and the first through fourth metatarsals.[7] These fractures have a favorable natural history and are less likely to recur, fail to unite, or have a significant complication should they progress to complete fracture. A subset of stress fractures can present a high risk for progression to complete fracture, delayed union, or nonunion. Specific sites for this type of stress fracture are the femoral neck (tension side), the patella, the anterior cortex of the tibia, the medial malleolus, the talus, the tarsal navicular, the fifth metatarsal, and the great toe sesamoids. Tensile forces and the relative avascularity at the site of a stress-induced fracture often lead to poor healing.[6]

PRESENTING COMPLAINT

Early diagnosis may be difficult and requires a high index of suspicion because patients may present with an insidious onset of pain with no obvious history of trauma. This pain may settle with cessation of activity but then recur on restarting activity. Although the location of pain may not always correlate with the area of injury, tibial stress injuries typically cause vague pain in the lower leg and may radiate to the ankle or knee.

HISTORY OF PRESENTING COMPLAINT

The pain typically begins after a change in the usual activity regimen or an increase in its intensity. It is usually insidious in onset and related to activity; however, in some cases the severity of pain may limit or prevent activity. Some patients may experience it at night.

The commonly held belief is that these fractures are injuries sustained by long distance runners and military recruits. However, other activities have been implicated in the generation of tibial stress injuries, such as ballet, volleyball, rowing, basketball, athletics, and gymnastics.[9–15] The overriding impression from the most recent articles is that the diagnosis should be considered in all athletes and military recruits, particularly women,[16,17] because it does not seem to be related as specifically to runners as previously thought.

It is particularly important to gain a satisfactory history from the patient to identify any factors that may be contributing to the development of stress fractures. These factors should include any recent alterations in training regimen[18,19] or surface[19,20] and the age of the patient's footwear.[18] A detailed menstrual history should be taken from women, including age at menarche,[21] any history of menstrual disturbance,[17,21–25] and contraceptive use.[22] It is also important to obtain a detailed history of the patient's dietary intake and any history of disordered eating.[26] Vitamin D deficiency is a potent cause of stress fractures and a rapidly increasingly diagnosed problem.[27]

PHYSICAL EXAMINATION

The presentation may be variable as is the physical examination. The examination begins with observation of the patient while entering the examination room. For stress fractures that have progressed, patients will often have a limp: a typical antalgic gait. Swelling may be found in the lower leg but this is not always present. The area of maximal tenderness is often easier to assess when compared with other stress fractures because of the subcutaneous nature of the tibia. With runners, this corresponds to the junction of the middle and distal thirds of the tibia; with military recruits, the proximal third tibia is involved, and with ballet dancers, the middle third tibia is a frequent site.[28,29] The muscle size, tone, and strength are usually unaffected by the stress reaction or fracture. Because the tibia is a long, subcutaneous bone, deep palpation of the involved area, if tolerated by the patient, may discover a stress fracture callus, or soft tissue swelling.[30] Also, percussion tenderness or a tuning fork[31] at a distance from the involved site may reproduce the patient's symptoms. Provocative tests may elicit pain at the appropriate site. These provocative tests may involve activities as simple as walking down the hallway or even running in place. Examination of the knee and hip reveals full, painless motion.

IMAGING STUDIES

Initial imaging of the tibia is usually undertaken using plain radiographs looking for radiolucent lines, cortical disruption, periosteal reaction, or early formation of callus. It is important to look for the "dreaded black line" that has been associated with the high-risk anterior cortex fracture. However, only 10% of these injuries demonstrate changes on plain radiograph at 1 week.[2] Periosteal bone formation is at its most prominent at 6 weeks.[32]

Technetium bone scans and MRI are the 2 modalities that are able to demonstrate the early changes seen in stress fractures. Because of its high sensitivity, bone scanning has been considered the gold standard for some time and is able to demonstrate the spectrum of changes within the bone that lead to development of stress reactions or fractures.[33,34] The sensitivity has been shown to be 84% to 100% within 3 days of symptoms.[35] However, despite its high sensitivity, bone scintigraphy lacks specificity because infection, osteonecrosis, and tumors can all mimic stress injury. Also, because the uptake can persist for months after clinical healing, bone scans are not as useful in follow-up care. The combination of computed tomographic (CT) scanning with a bone scan (single-photon emission CT) has added value to the bone scan.

MRI is extremely sensitive in the detection of soft tissue, bone, and marrow changes associated with stress injuries. It allows depiction of abnormalities weeks before the development of a radiographic lesion and has comparable sensitivity and superior specificity to scintigraphy.[36] In addition to bony changes, it also details information about the surrounding muscular or ligamentous insults associated with or responsible for the symptoms.[37] Kiuru and colleagues[38] have described a grading system based on the MRI appearance (**Table 1**).

The article by Arendt and Griffiths[39] describes a grading system for stress injuries, which takes into consideration the plain radiographic, scintigraphic, and MRI findings; from this, they make recommendations on return to sport based on these grades (**Table 2**). The same authors then followed up 10 years of using the grading scheme and return-to-play protocol in a subsequent article demonstrating a predictable return to play in these athletes.[40]

MANAGEMENT

Once the diagnosis of a tibial shaft stress reaction or stress fracture has been made, it is important for these injuries to be managed appropriately.

Several basic principles were outlined in the review by Raasch and Hergan in 2006 on the fundamentals of treatment of stress fractures[41]; first one must understand why the injury occurred in the first instance by considering the extrinsic and intrinsic factors that may have contributed to the injury. The extrinsic factors include the training regimen, equipment, and nutritional habits of the patient, whereas the intrinsic factors include anatomic variations, such as limb length discrepancies, muscle endurance, and hormonal/bone metabolism factors. Many of these factors will be picked up during the detailed history and the time spent during rehabilitation should also focus on these underlying factors to prevent recurrence.

Nonoperative Management

Following the diagnosis of tibial stress fracture from the history, physical examination, and imaging modalities, a treatment program needs to be commenced. The more common tibial stress fracture that occurs on the posteromedial aspect of the tibia usually responds to a period of rest followed by gradual resumption of activities. As alluded to earlier in the history, it is important to identify and modify any risk factors at this stage. Training regimen and footwear are easily correctable. Gait analysis and retraining may also play a role as biomechanical studies have demonstrated differences in those runners who sustain tibial stress fractures against matched controls.[42–46]

Addressing any nutritional, hormonal, or other medical abnormalities is essential in the promotion of fracture healing. Female patients, particularly athletes and dancers, need to be evaluated for eating disorders, amenorrhea, or oligomenorrhea and decreased bone density. Replacing estrogen returns the female athlete to a normal menstrual state and may improve bone mineral density given time.

Table 1	
Magnetic resonance imaging grading of stress injuries by Kiuru et al, 2004	
Grade	**MRI Findings**
I	Endosteal edema
II	Periosteal and endosteal edema
III	Muscle, periosteal, and endosteal edema
IV	Fracture line
V	Callus at the endosteal and/or periosteal surface of cortical bone

Table 2 Protocol based on MRI grading by Arendt and Griffiths, 1997	
Grade 1	3 wk rest
Grade 2	3–6 wk rest
Grade 3	12–16 wk rest
Grade 4	>16 wk rest

Definitive treatment protocols are based on the concept of the low-risk and high-risk fractures. The typical posteromedial stress fracture is considered lower risk, whereas the anterior (dreaded black line) stress fractures are considered higher risk. Low-risk fractures respond to rest for 2 to 6 weeks, with progressive return to activities. If the athlete is pain-free after a period of rest, then low-impact activities, such as biking and swimming, may be initiated. A graduated reintroduction of higher impact activities can be introduced while the patient remains asymptomatic. This process can take several months. If symptoms return, then the athlete may need to decrease activities again. Most posteromedial stress fractures heal in 1 to 2 months, but the average return to play is 3 to 4 months. Not all of these so-called low-risk fractures, however, respond to rest.

Weight-bearing status during the rest period comes down to clinical judgment. Intuitively, reducing the weight-bearing status to either non-weight-bearing or partial-weight-bearing, to decrease the force on the tibia seems sensible; however, there is no evidence showing that weight-bearing status affects the rate of healing. The use of pneumatic braces during this period has been studied. In one study, a small number of athletes were able to continue to compete with the pneumatic brace, and 11 of 13 became asymptomatic within 1 month despite the continued strain on the tibia.[47] Swenson and colleagues[48] demonstrated that those who wore pneumatic leg braces healed significantly more quickly when compared with those managed with rest alone. This demonstration was considered as part of a 2005 Cochrane review, which included this study and 2 others. There was some evidence from 3 small treatment trials that support of the injured leg in a pneumatic brace seemed to allow a return to training activity and thus a quicker rehabilitation. However, there were several flaws and confounding variables within the study designs.[49]

Operative Management

Operative intervention is usually reserved for those fractures that fail to respond to nonoperative management with rest and rehabilitation. These fractures often develop a chronic appearance that is visible on plain radiographs with sclerosis, cyst formation, and the dreaded black line. There are also some who advocate early fracture fixation in high-level athletes to decrease the time lost from their specific sport, assuming that return to play will be sooner.[50] **Figs. 1–3** demonstrate the preoperative and postoperative images of a UK-based Football Association Premiership footballer of African origin.

The surgical interventions that have been described for these fractures have been either drilling, with or without bone grafting, or intramedullary fixation. The basis of the drilling and bone grafting intervention is the concept that the chronic stress fracture acts like a pseudarthrosis[51]; therefore, by resecting the chronic fibrous material and stimulating the surrounding bone to act like a fresh fracture, the local biology becomes more favorable for healing.[52,53]

Intramedullary fixation is used to stabilize the fracture and provide a better mechanical environment for potential fracture healing by altering the biomechanical environment, load sharing, and stabilizing the fracture.[54,55]

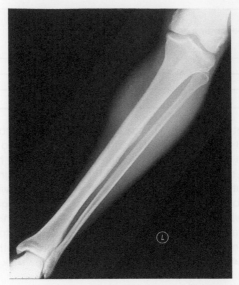

Fig. 1. Anteroposterior radiograph showing stress fracture. Periosteal reaction visible at the junction of proximal and middle thirds on lateral side.

Articles have been published on both techniques but are generally short cases series. Plasschaert and colleagues[56] published a case report in 1995 whereby conservative treatment, followed by drilling and then intramedullary fixation, had been tried for an anterior tibial stress fracture in a professional male ballet dancer, ultimately leading to union. A series by Miyamoto and colleagues[57] in 2009 described both

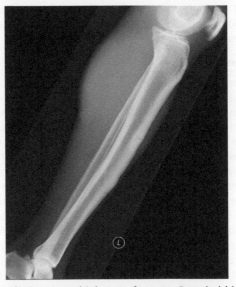

Fig. 2. Lateral radiograph showing tibial stress fracture. Dreaded black line visible at the same point as the periosteal reaction on the anterior cortex.

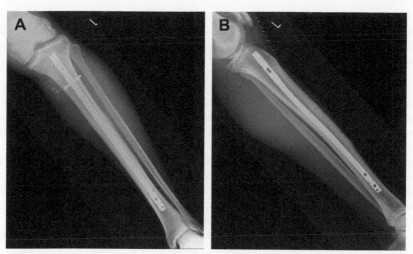

Fig. 3. (*A, B*) Postoperative anteroposterior and lateral radiographs following intramedullary nailing. Deliberately short intramedullary nail to decrease stress riser around ankle. Well-buried proximal end of nail to prevent irritation around the knee.

surgical options being used in refractory tibial stress fractures in elite ballet dancers, allowing all to return to dance with minimal morbidity.

Most surgeons now favor reamed intramedullary nailing because it allows redistribution of tibial loading and direct stimulation of healing by reaming.

There are technical aspects worth considering in athletes. The surgeon should consider medial parapatellar introduction of the nail to the proximal tibia rather than violate the patellar tendon, which is so vulnerable in an athlete. To avoid irritation of the distal patellar tendon, the proximal end of the nail should be buried well beneath the proximal cortical bone, and an end-cap for the nail used. If good diaphyseal contact occurs with the nail on either side of the fracture or at least distally, distal locking screws may be avoided so reducing the need for removal of metalwork before return to play. Postoperatively the senior author uses ultrasound wave therapy (Exogen; TM Smith and Nephew, Milford, NH, USA); however, evidence for the value of this is not certain (see later in discussion).

Adjuvant Treatment Modalities

A review article by Carmont and colleagues[58] assessed the evidence for several additional therapies in the management of stress fractures. They could find no compelling evidence to advocate the use of oxygen therapy, bisphosphonates, growth factors, bone morphogenic proteins, recombinant parathyroid hormone, and ultrasound or magnetic field application, in keeping with the review article by Young and McAllister in regard to medical intervention or ultrasound usage.[59]

Although there is little compelling statistically significant evidence that these modalities may improve the time to healing of tibial stress fractures, the closing comments of Carmont and colleagues[58] reflect the pragmatic approach that needs to be taken, particularly when treating elite athletes. They state, "...The physical methods used are unlikely to delay healing and may be preferable to biological techniques in which the full implications of their use may not be fully understood. Many of these new techniques will be difficult to obtain and are expensive. Thus, during the healing phase, the athlete should focus on conventional methods of relative rest, analgesia, and rehabilitation. Although surgical stabilization involves iatrogenic trauma to the area, the pain related to surgery may well force the athlete to rest, thus promoting healing and recovery..."

Summary

Tibial stress fractures are rare events in the general population but are much more common in the athletic and military population. A high index of suspicion is required to ensure early diagnosis. Once suspicion is raised of the injury, a detailed history, focused examination, and the appropriate imaging modalities are required to make the diagnosis and commence a patient-tailored rehabilitation program. It is important to consider contributory factors, such as hormonal or dietary imbalances during this period, especially Vitamin D deficiency. In the event of delayed union of the fracture, surgical intervention may be required and this is commonly using drilling, with or without bone grafting, or intramedullary fixation.

In most cases, athletes with tibial stress fractures can expect to return to their previous level of competition if they are compliant with the treatment program.

STRESS FRACTURES OF THE MEDIAL MALLEOLUS
Introduction

Demographics and incidence
Medial malleolar stress fractures are comparatively rare with a reported incidence of 0.6% to 4% of all lower limb stress fractures.[60,61] They occur almost exclusively in high-demand athletic individuals participating in running, jumping, and high-impact repetitive sports such as gymnastics.[60,61] Shabat and colleagues[62] reviewed the literature, identifying 4 studies reporting 23 cases. Eighteen of the 23 cases were men and the mean age was 24 years (15–60). All were very active competitive in sports, except for a 60-year-old woman who participated in recreational sports and had increased her level of activity significantly.

Pathophysiology
Risk factors for a medial malleolar stress fracture can be divided into intrinsic and extrinsic factors. Extrinsic factors may be training errors, poor footwear, a sudden increase in activity, weight gain, and so on. Many intrinsic risk factors have been proposed but most are speculative. Orava and colleagues[63] and Giladi and colleagues[64] in their reviews of stress fractures noted a predisposition to fracture with narrow tibia, increased external hip rotation, forefoot varus, subtalar varus, limb length discrepancy, tibial varus, and pes cavus. Devas[65] reported the first 2 cases of medial malleolar stress fracture. Of the 2 cases, one had a significant varus deformity of the tibia.

This was challenged by Schils and colleagues,[66] who only had one case of malalignment in their series of 7 medial malleolar stress fractures, a patient with bilateral tibia varus who united with conservative treatment. Orava and colleagues[63] in their series of 8 fractures also noted no particular mechanical or alignment abnormality yet. Okada and colleagues[67] in their single case identified distal tibial varus as an important etiologic factor. Biomechanically, a varus malalignment must subject the medial malleolus to greater rotational and sheer force but this may not always be clinically significant.

Jowett and colleagues[68] reported the association of anterior distal tibial osteophytes with medial malleolar stress fractures. In their series of 5 cases, all of whom were professional athletes, significant anteromedial spurs were identified in each case. The authors think the spurs led to impingement in terminal dorsiflexion, causing significant rotational and sheer forces through the malleolus. Anterior spurs and osteophytes are common in athletes[69,70] and many are asymptomatic.[71] They can be subtle to detect on radiographs and MRI, particularly anteromedial lesions,[72] and CT scan is a much better investigator for this abnormality (**Fig. 4**). It is likely that earlier studies may have missed some of the impingement lesions because most patients did not have CT scans. All 5 cases had the spur arthroscopically removed and the fracture internally fixed with a 100% union rate at a mean of 10.2 weeks. All patients returned to their previous level of play.

Clinical presentation and examination
Patients typically present with a history of increasing training intensity or a change in activity or sport. Certain patients may report no change in their routine and training. High-impact running and jumping activities are the most commonly associated activities. Usually there is no history of trauma. The pain is initially poorly localized to the medial ankle and side of the leg and gradually worsens as the microfracture propagates into a true stress fracture. With progression of the fracture, pain may become more localized to the fracture site. As with most stress fractures, the pain is usually activity related and relieved by rest. Because of the frequent intra-articular extension, stiffness and swelling of the ankle may also be a feature.

On examination, varus malalignment may be obvious and the gait pattern may be disturbed. The ankle typically has a normal range of motion unless there is a significant effusion or anterior spur. Tenderness to deep palpation over the malleolus, in particular, where the malleolus meets the plafond anteriorly is very confirmatory and many cases have a degree of localized soft tissue edema. Passive deep dorsiflexion may elicit the pain.

Diagnosis

Weight-bearing radiographs may reveal a fracture line in only 30% of cases.[72] These fracture lines are usually more chronic cases, with a longer duration of symptoms of

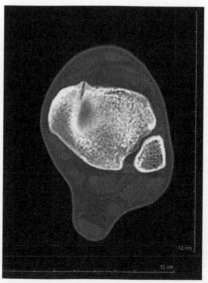

Fig. 4. Axial CT demonstrating fracture with associated anterior tibial spur.

4 to 6 weeks. Complete displacement of the malleolus is uncommon but is reported[69,70] and may result from neglected and undertreated cases. When a fracture line is present, it is vertically or obliquely orientated sometimes with associated small, well-circumscribed lytic lesions or cysts. Regional osteopenia, callus, sclerosis, or isolated cysts are other positive findings.[73] Cystic lesions are thought to be the result of bone resorption following local microfracture.[7]

Positive clinical findings and history together with negative radiographs warrant further imaging. Radionucleotide bone scan has been the modality of choice because of its almost 100% sensitivity. Radionucleotide bone scan is being replaced by MRI because it is as sensitive but also more specific (**Fig. 5**). False positive bone scans range from 13% to 24%.[73,74] MRI is also more accurate in precise anatomic localization of the fracture and in differentiating fracture from stress response. The typical MRI findings are a vertical linear decreased T1-weighted signal at the plafond-malleolus junction. Short tau inversion recovery sequences may reveal early stress fracture as increased signal, indicating edema and hemorrhage. Later there is a linear area of decreased signal on T2 imaging with increased surrounding bone marrow signal (**Fig. 6**).[75]

Fine-cut CT is less sensitive than MRI and bone scintigraphy at diagnosing fractures. It is a good tool in defining fracture configuration and local osseous anatomy (**Fig. 7**), particularly if a fracture and associated cysts are visible on radiographs, which can be helpful with surgical planning and also in identifying anterior spurs and osteophytes, which may warrant arthroscopic removal before fixation.

Treatment

There is little controversy that displaced fractures need an open reduction and internal fixation. These diplaced fractures are the minority of cases and the treatment options may need to be individualized to the particular patient for undisplaced fractures. Treatment depends on several factors, as follows:

1. The presence of a fracture line, cyst, or local osteopoenia on the radiographs.
2. Displacement of the fracture.

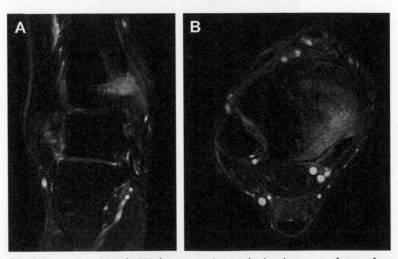

Fig. 5. (*A, B*) Coronal and axial MRI demonstrating early development of stress fracture of medial malleolus.

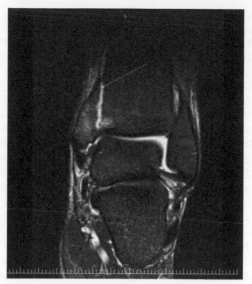

Fig. 6. Coronal MRI with *red arrow* demonstrating stress fracture through medial malleolus.

3. Level of sports or athletic participation.
4. Timing of the injury (in-season vs off-season).

Most patients who sustain this injury play a sport; many of whom may be competing at a high level. The time away from sport and participation may have serious personal and economic consequences for the individual and team or club.

There is a lack of good evidence to support either surgical or nonsurgical management, but certain factors may help make the decision for the surgeon and the patient. Because of the rarity of these fractures, case series and case reports must be relied on to shape the practice because no comparable studies with control groups exist.

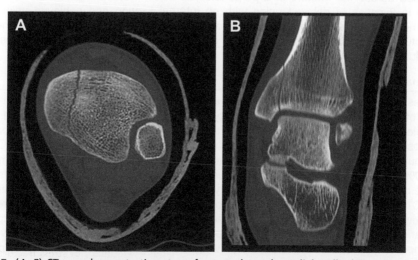

Fig. 7. (*A, B*) CT scan demonstrating stress fracture through medial malleolus.

Shabat and colleagues[62] reviewed 4 case studies involving 23 fractures and compared the time to return to sport after both surgical and nonsurgical treatment. Unfortunately the studies and treatments reviewed were not standardized and return to sports was not documented in all cases, resulting in weak evidence. There was a trend for the surgically treated group to have a faster return to sports in those patients whose return to sport was recorded (4.5 weeks vs 7 weeks). Union was achieved faster in the surgically treated patients (4.2 months vs 6.7 months). Reider and coworkers[76] reported the nonunion of a stress fracture treated conservatively with cast immobilization for 6 weeks and a gradual return to activity. The nonunion required bone grafting and a prolonged period of protected weight-bearing. Orava and colleagues[63] treated 7 of 8 patients with cast immobilization and prolonged avoidance of impact activity (5 months). Two patients required drilling of the fracture site for delayed union. One patient received an AO compression screw (Synthes, West Chester, PA, USA) for a displaced fracture. The mean time to return to sports participation was 7 months. Shelbourne and colleagues[77] treated 6 medial malleolar stress fractures, 3 surgically with compression screws and 3 nonsurgically with immobilization and non-weight-bearing for 6 weeks. If a fracture line was visible on radiographs, the patient had surgery, and if not, conservative treatment with a gradual return to activity was instigated. The results were similar with return to full activity for both groups at 6 to 8 weeks. Jowett and colleagues[68] achieved union in all 5 patients with compression screws together with removal of the anteromedial spur arthroscopically. They did not document when their patients returned to sports but all did reach their preinjury level postsurgery.

The principle of treating a stress fracture is to relieve the stress by resting the limb or patient, allowing the bone to heal. Some authors advocate conservative management of medial malleolar stress fractures with a period of immobilization and a slow return to weight-bearing and impact having shown good results in their series.[66,73,77,78] Immobilization of the ankle results in rapid calf atrophy and ankle stiffness, ultimately delaying return to athletic performance. Pro-surgical authors argue that internal fixation allows the patient to maintain ankle motion as the internal fixation stabilizes the malleolus, allowing a faster return to activity.[62,68,76,79] The surgical techniques used in the literature are either open or percutaneous compression screws placed across the fracture in a perpendicular fashion. Orava[63] drilled the fracture site in 2 cases of delayed union with no internal fixation and achieved union at 10 months. The use of osteobiologics and bone grafting has not been studied in these fractures but may have a role. Bone grafting has been successful in cases of nonunion.[76]

Summary

Stress fractures of the medial malleolus are not common. They typically occur in the athletic population manifesting as activity-related pain around the medial side of the ankle with or without ankle swelling and stiffness. Axial malalignment, anterior spurs, or osteophytes and torsional forces are etiologic factors in their development. Only about 30% of fractures are visible on radiographs but bone scan and MRI have almost 100% sensitivity in diagnosing the fracture. Treatment should be guided by the fracture displacement, level of patient activity, and evidence of a fracture on radiographs or CT scan. The surgical technique of choice is the placement of compression screws followed by non-weight-bearing for 2 weeks and then a gradual return to full weight-bearing, maintaining range of motion throughout. Conservative treatment is a 4-week period of immobilization and protected weight-bearing with a slow return to impact activity. See **Fig. 8** for treatment algorithm.

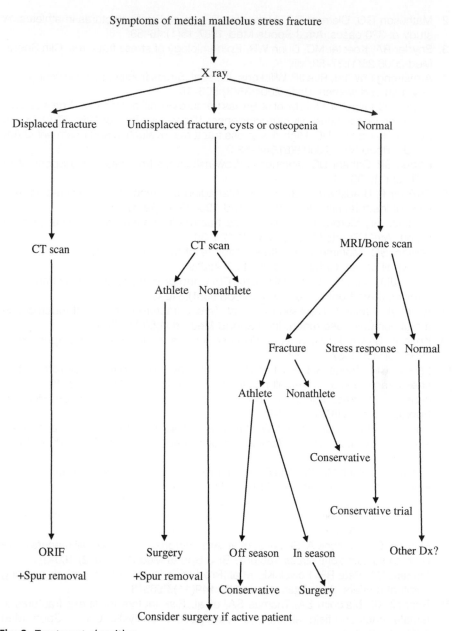

Fig. 8. Treatment algorithm.

REFERENCES

1. Court-Brown C, Caesar BC. The epidemiology of fractures (part 1) overview of epidemiology. In: Buchloz RW, Heckman JD, Court-Brown CM, editors. Rockwood and Green's fractures in adults. 6th edition. Philadelphia: Lippincott, Williams and Wilkins; 2006. p. 95–113.

2. Matheson GO, Clement DB, McKenzie DC, et al. Stress fractures in athletes. A study of 320 cases. Am J Sports Med 1987;15(1):46–58.
3. Snyder RA, Koester MC, Dunn WR. Epidemiology of stress fractures. Clin Sports Med 2006;25(1):37–52, viii.
4. Armstrong DW 3rd, Rue JP, Wilckens JH, et al. Stress fracture injury in young military men and women. Bone 2004;35(3):806–16.
5. Milgrom C, Giladi M, Stein M, et al. Stress fractures in military recruits. A prospective study showing an unusually high incidence. J Bone Joint Surg Br 1985;67(5):732–5.
6. Boden BP, Osbahr DC. High-risk stress fractures: evaluation and treatment. J Am Acad Orthop Surg 2000;8(6):344–53.
7. Boden BP, Osbahr DC, Jimenez C. Low-risk stress fractures. Am J Sports Med 2001;29(1):100–11.
8. Brukner P, Bradshaw C, Bennell K. Managing common stress fractures: let risk level guide treatment. Phys Sportsmed 1998;26(8):39–47.
9. Martinez SF, Murphy GA. Tibial stress fracture in a male ballet dancer: a case report. Am J Sports Med 2005;33(1):124–30.
10. Tejwani SG, Motamedi AR. Stress fracture of the tibial tubercle in a collegiate volleyball player. Orthopedics 2004;27(2):219–22.
11. Losito JM, Laird RC, Alexis MR, et al. Tibial and proximal fibular stress fracture in a rower. J Am Podiatr Med Assoc 2003;93(4):340–3.
12. Israeli A, Ganel A, Blankstein A, et al. Stress fracture of the tibial tuberosity in a high jumper: case report. Int J Sports Med 1984;5(6):299–300.
13. Khan K, Brown J, Way S, et al. Overuse injuries in classical ballet. Sports Med 1995;19(5):341–57.
14. Larson CM, Traina SM, Fischer DA, et al. Recurrent complete proximal tibial stress fracture in a basketball player. Am J Sports Med 2005;33(12):1914–7.
15. Jensen JE. Stress fracture in the world class athlete: a case study. Med Sci Sports Exerc 1998;30(6):783–7.
16. Rauh MJ, Macera CA, Trone DW, et al. Epidemiology of stress fracture and lower-extremity overuse injury in female recruits. Med Sci Sports Exerc 2006;38(9):1571–7.
17. Shaffer RA, Rauh MJ, Brodine SK, et al. Predictors of stress fracture susceptibility in young female recruits. Am J Sports Med 2006;34(1):108–15.
18. Gardner LI Jr, Dziados JE, Jones BH, et al. Prevention of lower extremity stress fractures: a controlled trial of a shock absorbent insole. Am J Public Health 1988;78(12):1563–7.
19. Milgrom C, Finestone A, Segev S, et al. Are overground or treadmill runners more likely to sustain tibial stress fracture? Br J Sports Med 2003;37(2):160–3.
20. Macera CA, Pate RR, Powell KE, et al. Predicting lower-extremity injuries among habitual runners. Arch Intern Med 1989;149(11):2565–8.
21. Bennell KL, Malcolm SA, Thomas SA, et al. Risk factors for stress fractures in female track-and-field athletes: a retrospective analysis. Clin J Sport Med 1995;5(4):229–35.
22. Barrow GW, Saha S. Menstrual irregularity and stress fractures in collegiate female distance runners. Am J Sports Med 1988;16(3):209–16.
23. Brukner P, Bennell K. Stress fractures in female athletes. Diagnosis, management and rehabilitation. Sports Med 1997;24(6):419–29.
24. Korpelainen R, Orava S, Karpakka J, et al. Risk factors for recurrent stress fractures in athletes. Am J Sports Med 2001;29(3):304–10.
25. Tomten SE, Falch JA, Birkeland KI, et al. Bone mineral density and menstrual irregularities. A comparative study on cortical and trabecular bone structures

in runners with alleged normal eating behavior. Int J Sports Med 1998;19(2): 92–7.

26. Kadel NJ, Teitz CC, Kronmal RA. Stress fractures in ballet dancers. Am J Sports Med 1992;20(4):445–9.

27. McClung JP, Karl JP. Vitamin D and stress fracture: the contribution of vitamin D receptor gene polymorphisms. Nutr Rev 2010;68(6):365–9.

28. Hershman EB, Mailly T. Stress fractures. Clin Sports Med 1990;9(1):183–214.

29. Meyer SA, Saltzman CL, Albright JP. Stress fractures of the foot and leg. Clin Sports Med 1993;12(2):395–413.

30. Sterling JC, Edelstein DW, Calvo RD, et al. Stress fractures in the athlete. Diagnosis and management. Sports Med 1992;14(5):336–46.

31. Lesho EP. Can tuning forks replace bone scans for identification of tibial stress fractures? Mil Med 1997;162(12):802–3.

32. Knapp TP, Garrett WE Jr. Stress fractures: general concepts. Clin Sports Med 1997;16(2):339–56.

33. Wilcox JR Jr, Moniot AL, Green JP. Bone scanning in the evaluation of exercise-related stress injuries. Radiology 1977;123(3):699–703.

34. Zwas ST, Elkanovitch R, Frank G. Interpretation and classification of bone scintigraphic findings in stress fractures. J Nucl Med 1987;28(4):452–7.

35. Couture CJ, Karlson KA. Tibial stress injuries: decisive diagnosis and treatment of 'shin splints'. Phys Sportsmed 2002;30(6):29–36.

36. Datir AP. Stress-related bone injuries with emphasis on MRI. Clin Radiol 2007; 62(9):828–36.

37. Spitz DJ, Newberg AH. Imaging of stress fractures in the athlete. Radiol Clin North Am 2002;40(2):313–31.

38. Kiuru MJ, Pihlajamaki HK, Ahovuo JA. Bone stress injuries. Acta Radiol 2004; 45(3):317–26.

39. Arendt EA, Griffiths HJ. The use of MR imaging in the assessment and clinical management of stress reactions of bone in high-performance athletes. Clin Sports Med 1997;16(2):291–306.

40. Arendt E, Agel J, Heikes C, et al. Stress injuries to bone in college athletes: a retrospective review of experience at a single institution. Am J Sports Med 2003;31(6): 959–68.

41. Raasch WG, Hergan DJ. Treatment of stress fractures: the fundamentals. Clin Sports Med 2006;25(1):29–36, vii.

42. Crowell HP, Davis IS. Gait retraining to reduce lower extremity loading in runners. Clin Biomech (Bristol, Avon) 2011;26(1):78–83.

43. Haris Phuah A, Schache AG, Crossley KM, et al. Sagittal plane bending moments acting on the lower leg during running. Gait Posture 2010;31(2):218–22.

44. Milner CE, Davis IS, Hamill J. Free moment as a predictor of tibial stress fracture in distance runners. J Biomech 2006;39(15):2819–25.

45. Milner CE, Hamill J, Davis I. Are knee mechanics during early stance related to tibial stress fracture in runners? Clin Biomech (Bristol, Avon) 2007;22(6): 697–703.

46. Zifchock RA, Davis I, Hamill J. Kinetic asymmetry in female runners with and without retrospective tibial stress fractures. J Biomech 2006;39(15):2792–7.

47. Dickson TB Jr, Kichline PD. Functional management of stress fractures in female athletes using a pneumatic leg brace. Am J Sports Med 1987;15(1):86–9.

48. Swenson EJ Jr, DeHaven KE, Sebastianelli WJ, et al. The effect of a pneumatic leg brace on return to play in athletes with tibial stress fractures. Am J Sports Med 1997;25(3):322–8.

49. Rome K, Handoll HH, Ashford R. Interventions for preventing and treating stress fractures and stress reactions of bone of the lower limbs in young adults. Cochrane Database Syst Rev 2005;(2):CD000450.
50. Barrick EF, Jackson CB. Prophylactic intramedullary fixation of the tibia for stress fracture in a professional athlete. J Orthop Trauma 1992;6(2):241–4.
51. Rolf C, Ekenman I, Tornqvist H, et al. The anterior stress fracture of the tibia: an atrophic pseudoarthosis? Scand J Med Sci Sports 1997;7(4):249–52.
52. Green NE, Rogers RA, Lipscomb AB. Nonunions of stress fractures of the tibia. Am J Sports Med 1985;13(3):171–6.
53. Orava S, Karpakka J, Hulkko A, et al. Diagnosis and treatment of stress fractures located at the mid-tibial shaft in athletes. Int J Sports Med 1991;12(4):419–22.
54. Chang PS, Harris RM. Intramedullary nailing for chronic tibial stress fractures. A review of five cases. Am J Sports Med 1996;24(5):688–92.
55. Varner KE, Younas SA, Lintner DM, et al. Chronic anterior midtibial stress fractures in athletes treated with reamed intramedullary nailing. Am J Sports Med 2005;33(7):1071–6.
56. Plasschaert VF, Johansson CG, Micheli LJ. Anterior tibial stress fracture treated with intramedullary nailing: a case report. Clin J Sport Med 1995;5(1):58–61 [discussion: 61–2].
57. Miyamoto RG, Dhotar HS, Rose DJ, et al. Surgical treatment of refractory tibial stress fractures in elite dancers: a case series. Am J Sports Med 2009;37(6):1150–4.
58. Carmont M, Mei-Dan O, Bennell K. Stress fracture management: current classification and new healing modalities. Oper Tech Sports Med 2009;17:9.
59. Young AJ, McAllister DR. Evaluation and treatment of tibial stress fractures. Clin Sports Med 2006;25(1):117–28, x.
60. Brukner P, Bradshaw C, Khan KM, et al. Stress fractures: a review of 180 cases. Clin J Sport Med 1996;6(2):85–9.
61. Iwamoto J, Takeda T. Stress fractures in athletes: review of 196 cases. J Orthop Sci 2003;8(3):273–8.
62. Shabat S, Sampson KB, Mann G, et al. Stress fractures of the medial malleolus–review of the literature and report of a 15-year-old elite gymnast. Foot Ankle Int 2002;23(7):647–50.
63. Orava S, Karpakka J, Taimela S, et al. Stress fracture of the medial malleolus. J Bone Joint Surg Am 1995;77(3):362–5.
64. Giladi M, Milgrom C, Simkin A, et al. Stress fractures. Identifiable risk factors. Am J Sports Med 1991;19(6):647–52.
65. Devas MB. Stress fractures of the tibia in athletes or shin soreness. J Bone Joint Surg Br 1958;40(2):227–39.
66. Schils JP, Andrish JT, Piraino DW, et al. Medial malleolar stress fractures in seven patients: review of the clinical and imaging features. Radiology 1992;185(1):219–21.
67. Okada K, Senma S, Abe E, et al. Stress fractures of the medial malleolus: a case report. Foot Ankle Int 1995;16(1):49–52.
68. Jowett AJ, Birks CL, Blackney MC. Medial malleolar stress fracture secondary to chronic ankle impingement. Foot Ankle Int 2008;29(7):716–21.
69. McMurray T. Footballers ankle. J Bone Joint Surg Br 1950;32:68–9.
70. Ferkel RD, Scranton PE Jr. Arthroscopy of the ankle and foot. J Bone Joint Surg Am 1993;75(8):1233–42.
71. Massada JL. Ankle overuse injuries in soccer players. Morphological adaptation of the talus in the anterior impingement. J Sports Med Phys Fitness 1991;31(3):447–51.

72. Steinbronn DJ, Bennett GL, Kay DB. The use of magnetic resonance imaging in the diagnosis of stress fractures of the foot and ankle: four case reports. Foot Ankle Int 1994;15(2):80–3.
73. Sherbondy PS, Sebastianelli WJ. Stress fractures of the medial malleolus and distal fibula. Clin Sports Med 2006;25(1):129–37, x.
74. Stafford SA, Rosenthal DI, Gebhardt MC, et al. MRI in stress fracture. AJR Am J Roentgenol 1986;147(3):553–6.
75. Timins ME. MR imaging of the foot and ankle. Foot Ankle Clin 2000;5(1):83–101, vi.
76. Reider B, Falconiero R, Yurkofsky J. Nonunion of a medial malleolus stress fracture. A case report. Am J Sports Med 1993;21(3):478–81.
77. Shelbourne KD, Fisher DA, Rettig AC, et al. Stress fractures of the medial malleolus. Am J Sports Med 1988;16(1):60–3.
78. Devas MB, Sweetnam DR. Runner's fracture. Practitioner 1958;180(1077):340–2.
79. Kor A, Saltzman AT, Wempe PD. Medial malleolar stress fractures. Literature review, diagnosis, and treatment. J Am Podiatr Med Assoc 2003;93(4):292–7.

Phases of Rehabilitation

Bryan English, MB ChB, FFSEM

KEYWORDS

- Rehabilitation • Athlete • Orthopedics

KEY POINTS

- Control of tissue swelling is required before commencement of rehabilitation.
- High-level athletes require rehabilitation of the whole patient before return to sports.
- Injury prevention programs must be in place before returning to sports; the highest risk factor for further ankle injury is a previous injury.

INTRODUCTION

The definition of rehabilitation is, "To restore to useful life, as through therapy and education. To restore to good condition, operation or capacity.[1]"

Rehabilitation is easy to do badly and difficult to do well. A technically excellent operative procedure can be undermined by poor rehabilitation, and an average procedure can be complimented by expert rehabilitation.

Rehabilitation is performed by a variety of specialists, and the closer they work as a team, the more successful the end result. Rehabilitation is not the focus of one practitioner. It may be mainly performed by one practitioner, but the construction, judgment, and case management of the process must have input from several professionals with differing areas of training and expertise. However, someone must take responsibility for the whole process, and the most appropriate person within a large medical team would be the physician with training and expertise within this field.

Many ways exist in which to rehabilitate a medical problem. In relation to orthopedics, this functional rehabilitation can fall into 7 categories;

1. Decrease pain and swelling
2. Achieve full range of movement and flexibility
3. Achieve full power and endurance
4. Achieve top levels of proprioception and coordination
5. Achieve previous level of agility and skill
6. Return to full training, with prevention
7. Return to play

Following some form of structure in rehabilitation is important. Structure that is preferably, but not essentially, backed with some form of science/evidence gives the

The Fortius Clinic, 17 Fitzhardinge Street, London, W1H 6EQ, UK
E-mail address: bryan.english@btinternet.com

Foot Ankle Clin N Am 18 (2013) 357–367
http://dx.doi.org/10.1016/j.fcl.2013.02.011
1083-7515/13/$ – see front matter © 2013 Published by Elsevier Inc.
foot.theclinics.com

patient and the rehabilitation team confidence and reassurance that all is going to be well. Education of the staff and the patient through the process is important, because each patient brings personal challenges. Previous history, expectations, operative success, and time availability for rehabilitation (before necessity of return to work) will lead to a case-by-case personal rehabilitation plan rather than a heavy protocol-based prescription. Constant review of the success/failure of the rehabilitation process is healthy to avoid following a path that may lead to failure. For this reason, measurements, such as range of movement of a joint, heart response to exercise, maximal speed, and ability to decelerate, can be recorded to show the rehabilitation team and the patient that progress is being made. Return to full training criteria can be created as target setting to provide a focus for motivation, and standard setting for those performing the assessments and treatments.

Assessment of the rehabilitation phases can encompass state of the art scientific evaluation, such as high-speed video analysis, accelerometers, and global positioning system (GPS) satellite data. However, it can also be performed using a stopwatch and some sticks in the ground. In other words, the process should be creative and imaginative for the practitioner. The process should be enjoyable, possible, and affordable for the patient.

To the reader, the author makes a small apology that the text is not illustrated. The author believes that rehabilitation is a functional process and is best demonstrated by video. Still images lead to misconceptions, which is why the written word is preferred.

PHASE 1: DECREASE THE PAIN AND SWELLING

After an injury or operation, the main focus is to keep swelling to a minimum, with the hope that this will also minimize pain. Pain and swelling will prevent the progress towards phase 2. Many methods are available to alleviate swelling; however, compression, cooling, and elevation seem to be the mainstays of treatment. One should also include "decreased function," because early lack of swelling and pain can lead to complacency, causing the patient to want to begin moving to "try it out." The importance of rest and recovery, even if just for 48 hours depending on the case, can be very productive, and the patient should be educated regarding why this is important. If the surgery was elective, then the hope is that the patient took steps to create a support network to assist in the rehabilitation phase when at home (because returning home as soon as is possible is beneficial to all).[2,3]

Gentle active resisted muscle activation is possible at this stage, and can be induced by electrical activation, to avoid the muscle-damaging effect of pain and swelling.

Aquatic therapy is an excellent modality to ease swelling and pain because of the compressive effect of water and the beneficial effect of minimal movement in deep water.[4-11] Naturally there may be anxiety with regard to wound protection; however, this anxiety should lead to expertise in wound protection and management, and aquatic therapy in these circumstances should not be contraindicated, because no evidence indicates that well-maintained pool chemistry should cause a problem (especially when the wound can be covered with waterproof dressing).[12,13]

Analgesia has its place at this stage to decrease inflammation and allow the patient to become more mobile and, importantly, adopt as normal a gait as possible as early as possible.

Manual therapy/effleurage is a useful way to make patients feel that they are being looked after (do not underestimate the power of this), and gentle passive mobilization will start to alleviate patients' fear that movement will cause pain. The manual therapist will get a feeling of the degree of swelling, warmth and range of the injured area, and the reactivity of the contractile tissues. This hands-on knowledge is valuable in determining progression or regression in this initial crucial phase. Wound breakdown, bleeding, and infection can be easily avoided with care and diligence from experienced professionals. An overzealous rehabilitation team or overambitious impatient patient can disturb the healing phase at this stage and send the plan completely off-course. Leadership and guidance at this stage is a priority to support those responsible for the success or failure of rehabilitation. The hope is that good communication between all parties will see the patient through phase 1 as soon as possible without fear and with a positive expectation of phase 2 (which naturally overlaps a with phase 1 on a case-by-case basis).

Can Phase 1 Be Measured? Yes

Swelling can be measured with limb girth daily. Pain can be measured using many methods, such as the visual analog scale (VAS).

PHASE 2: ACHIEVE FULL RANGE OF MOVEMENT AND FLEXIBILITY

The range of movement of the joints and contractile tissues involved (proximal and distal to the injury) should be encouraged as soon as possible. Fear and pain should not interfere unless a specific reason exists to restrict movement. Increased range can be encouraged through passive and active movements of the joints and soft tissues. Both passive and active movements should be observed, documented, and, where possible, measured with reproducibility. Methods for measurements should be standardized and discussed by the rehabilitation team to encourage good intermeasurer reliability, while recognizing that intratester testing may be ideal.

Knowledge of range of movement before injury is beneficial, which is why annual musculoskeletal screening/profiling is beneficial in sport. However, the contralateral limb is also a good comparison, with obvious assumptions being made about preinjury symmetry.

The patient is often anxious in this phase and must be educated that increasing range is not often a pain-free process. Warming up the joint (applied heat or exercise) before the end range of movement can help. Cradling of the joint with experienced hands can provide reassurance during the passive movement phase. Active movements can be encouraged with the use of aquatic therapy along with many other tools, such as static cycling.

Daily measurement can provide a visual for the medical team and the patient, with goal setting providing a target. These measurements also act as a guide for whether the mobilization is being overdone (resulting in increased swelling and decreased range of movements, especially first thing in the morning).

Can Phase 2 Range of Movement Be Measured? Yes

Goniometers are still a useful tool to measure range of movement of a joint while recognizing that the range may be restricted because of issues such as swelling, tight soft tissues, pain, and bone.

Flexibility is less easy to measure, because these measurements tend to be more global than local. Ability to touch the toes with extended knees (for fear of using a rather clumsy example) covers movements of the spine, sacroiliac joints, hip, knee, and ankle, along with associated ligament, tendon, muscle, fascia, and neurovascular structures. However, this should not deter the medical team from addressing all of these structures to obtain full range of movement. The use of passive and active stretches, manual therapy, active resisted techniques (hold, contract, stretch), and techniques to decrease hypertonic tissue (heat, electrical therapy) can all be considered as part of the arsenal to create as much range as possible.[14]

Can Phase 2 Flexibility Be Measured? Yes

Knee to wall test, for example, can demonstrate flexibility of the calf muscle and/or deep flexors of the foot and ankle and range of movement of the ankle. The practitioner must determine whether this restriction is from the lack of range or of flexibility. These tests can be arranged for any joint and can be combined with range assessment.

The importance of experience in this phase cannot be underestimated. It is paramount to achieve good range early (extension after anterior cruciate surgery for example), with sympathy for the restriction and information provided from the tissues during the treatment process. Careful mobilization may indicate that the joint is just not ready for the range, because too much swelling, too much pain, or a defective surgical procedure is present. When dealing with living human tissue, one can "listen" to the structure rather than just mobilizing and forcing the restriction. This phase, like many of the others, can be individual. Some joints will respond well and the patient can accelerate through the process, whereas other joints will react and require more patience. Therefore, progression should be the target, and goal setting should not be hastened by unrealistic time schedules. Occasionally, "rest" for 48 hours can allow the joint to settle and follow a much more productive phase.

PHASE 3: ACHIEVE FULL POWER AND ENDURANCE

The overlap between phase 1 and 2 is marked. However, little overlap is seen between phase 2 and 3, because progress in phase 3 is limited and even switched off. For example, vastus medialis switches off with a knee effusion and, in the author's opinion, tibialis posterior switches off with an ankle effusion.[15,16] One cannot get the power back in these areas and exercise them to the full until one has gotten past phase 1 and 2 completely. In contrast, the early stages of phase 4 can be introduced in the mid stages of phase 3.

Power is a muscle's expression of full physiologic function, and is one of the most easily measured of the modalities (using instruments such as weights, scales, dynamometers, and isokinetic machines). The progress can easily be recorded to show maximal effort or exercise to fatigue (can the patient perform 10 lunges, for example) using scientific laboratory–based assessment and field testing of functional movement patterns.

Can Power Be Measured in Phase 3? Yes

Exercise is key in phase 3. Isometric and isotonic exercise are inexpensive and easy to perform as a self-management process, and can be performed with the joint isolated (eg, knee extension while sitting) or, as one may prefer, using the whole kinetic chain (eg, the standing jump). These movements can be measured and are repeatable and reliable.[17–21]

Can Endurance Be Measured in Phase 3? Yes

Repeated calf raises to fatigue can be measured; however, the quality of movement must be supervised. Repeated concentric loading at a certain speed can be accurately measured with an isokinetic machine. These tests can measure isolated endurance.

Whole-body endurance is also important at this stage and can be measured with lactate testing during treadmill running, for example (or through devising another exercise for a multidirectional athlete). Lactate testing involves sequential blood samples measuring the increase in body lactate as a response to increasing exercise. The less fit the individual, the quicker the body lactate increases. A less invasive way to measure fitness can be through field testing and observing heat rate response to a submaximal exercise (eg, the Yo-Yo intermittent recovery test).[22]

Whole-body endurance work is sometimes wrongly ignored in stage 3, more because of fear on the part of the practitioner than anything else. After passing phase 2, the patient should not be viewed as a fragile being that is going to break down. The injured area can be respected while the body performs heavy cardiovascular work.

The heart can be worked hard in the water, for example. Individuals can exercise in deep water in numerous ways to produce a significant cardiorespiratory challenge. The big muscle groups can be challenged with power repetitions to produce/reinforce range, power, and flexibility. The exercises can be designed to be entertaining to aid compliance, and the practitioner should ideally be of a physical state to participate and demonstrate the work to the patient (with intermittent breaks, such as head tennis in the water, for recovery).

A higher state of monitoring can involve the wearing of a heart rate monitor throughout the working day to obtain an estimate of cardiovascular "work done."

PHASE 4: ACHIEVE TO LEVELS OF PROPRIOCEPTION AND COORDINATION

Phase 4 is arguably the most important rehabilitation phase. The author's opinion is that phase 4 is easy to dismiss by the improving athlete eager to get to phase 5 and beyond. Phase 4 requires concentration and discipline from the practitioner and the patient. However, understanding human nature, the practitioner may wish to introduce aspects of phase 5 to provide a taste of things to come when phase 4 has been successfully mastered.

Phase 4 also allows the artistry and imagination of the practitioner to flourish. Using the discipline of balance, proprioception and coordination in a variety of ways to enable the patient to master body control, can be rewarding.

Movements that test and train proprioception and coordination must be diverse, challenging, entertaining, and relevant to the person's future activity, which helps with compliance.

A plethora of examples exist regarding how to do this work. One simple example is the hop–and–hold test, which can highlight deficiencies in patients who may notice the asymmetry with this basic movement (and therefore understand that phase 5 is not possible without being able to control function in phase 4).

This test can progress to different surfaces, such as sand or a trampoline. The complexity of the test can be heightened by asking the patient to catch a ball after landing the hold phase.[23–27]

The goal is to safely increase the complexity of the work that is being performed by the body continuously. The execution of the work must be good, otherwise the patient may be learning abnormal movement patterns that will be difficult to undo at a later stage. If the body learns highly complex tasks and performs these well, then the introduction of phase 5 will proceed safely.

Can Proprioception and Coordination Be Measured? Yes

Balancing and hop-and-hold tests can be visualized and videoed. The amount of sway can be measured on force platforms, as can the quality of foot strike and propulsive force (if one wishes to take these measurements into the biomechanics laboratory).

Revisiting phase 4 with the new challenge of different surfaces, such as sand and the trampoline, can lead to a higher level of function and increase the challenge for the patient and player.[28–32]

PHASE 5: ACHIEVE PREVIOUS LEVELS OF SKILL AND AGILITY

Phase 5 is the exciting phase at which patients begin to feel as though they are "nearly there." Therefore, it is a positive phase, but also a dangerous one. Some important skills remain to be learned during this phase.

Patients and players may now be under pressure to return to full activity because they are seen to be functioning at a high level. The player must begin to prepare to return to work. For example, after an injury to the ankle syndesmosis, at this phase the player has:

1. No ankle swelling or pain and good range of movement
2. Good power of the calf, deep flexors, peroneals, and thigh/buttock musculature, and the Yo-Yo test shows good cardiovascular endurance compared with previous testing
3. Basic proprioception and coordination in the water, sand, trampoline, and grass, showing symmetry

Therefore, the player must now:

1. Perform tasks relating to the sport, such as kicking, jumping, twisting, sprinting, and tackling
2. Perform these tasks with increasing load, such as with a heavier ball, greater speed of movement, and tighter angle of movement, and involving contact from other players or trainers
3. Repeat these tasks hundreds of times with precise execution and quality of movement to begin matching the demands of full training

By the time the patient leaves this phase, the rehabilitation team will know that the demands of full training have been met and no dramatic increase in demand will occur when they return to training.

If the player is working with a good quality rehabilitation, then this phase may cross-over daily with phase 6. During this phase, the player is allowed to participate in some, but not all, parts of training. This gradual return will help rehabilitation proceed with a mutual understating of limits among those involved and will allow the process to be tailored to the individual needs of the player.

Can Phase 5 Be Measured? Yes

Phase 5 can be measured, and many of these methods are used in phase 6 and discussed in the next section. The speed and movement of the individual can measured, and the quality of movement and agility can be seen on video or measured with accelerometers in the field. The accuracy of kicking a moving ball can be seen and felt by the rehabilitator. Although some of the skill-related work may be difficult to measure, a type of VAS exists for this form of work. The rehabilitator/trainer may mention that the quality of short ball striking is 10 of 10; however, the long ball striking is 8 of 10 for power and 6 of 10 for accuracy.

PHASE 6: RETURN TO FULL TRAINING WITH PREVENTION

Return to training criteria can be set in the initial stages of rehabilitation. These criteria may take several forms. For example, for a 75-year-old bowls player recovering from an ankle arthroscopy, these criteria may be:

1. Maximal ankle range compared with the normal side or an acceptable range
2. No swelling or pain

3. Ability to walk up and down stairs without pain
4. Ability to get out of a chair using both legs (separately)
5. Ability to perform crown green bowling for an hour
6. Understanding self-management strategies

Another example could be a professional football player recovering from the same operation, for whom the criteria may be:

1. Maximal joint range compared with the other side/preinjury range
2. No pain or swelling
3. Maximal isotonic/isokinetic power of lower leg musculature
4. Maximal jump test compared with previous measures (compare left vs. right)
5. Ability to perform hop-and-hold test with maximal proprioception/agility
6. Attain preinjury levels of number and quality of maximal accelerations and decelerations comparing right and left sides
7. Ability to manage striking a ball and endurance work on the grass for up to time spent in a normal training session
8. Accepting and complying with self-management work

These scenarios provide 2 brief examples of return–to-training criteria that may be used when a patient is ready to return to sport without support, but with the assurance that compliance with self-management strategies will be high.

Unrealistic and unreasonable demands are counterproductive and may lead to frustration and disappointment. Realistic goal-setting is important.

A visual display or chart can be used (similar to a VAS) to show how close to the target the patient has progressed over the previous days or weeks.

Can Phase 6 Be Measured? Yes

Technology offers a multitude of support to assess function of human movement. Scales, cameras, dynamometers, accelerometers, GPS systems, heart rate monitors, and stop watches are pieces of equipment to measure the most basic of human movements up to the most dynamic movements. These measurements are reproducible and can be collected and digitized to create a library of functional analysis. The process of the data and its application in relation to the clinician depends on the interest and education of the clinician. Reams of meaningless and difficult-to-apply data can cause a great loss of time and money. Data that are easy to apply can prevent a "nearly healed" injury from being overexposed or underexposed in the rehabilitation process.

Prevention is the great challenge when completing phase 6. Compliance requires education and understanding of the need for prevention.

For example, an arthritic ankle in a tennis player may require occasional assessment to monitor the range of movement of the joint and to encourage compliance with work to increase that range (if it is found to be quietly decreasing). Therefore, although it may be asymptomatic, the work on the range of movement may prevent other issues, such as a calf muscle tear.

Prevention also involves good recovery strategies (eg, nutrition, rest, sleep) and the avoidance of overexercise and underexercise. Cross-training (eg, a football player swimming or playing table tennis) and executing good movement patterns (eg, the hop–and-hold test) should also be part of the discipline of injury and illness avoidance.

Prevention is difficult to measure within a small number of people and over a short time, because the only measure is the percentage of injury recurrence (which is multifactorial). Although difficult to measure, the hope is that patient education will lead to individuals assuming responsibility for self-management (similar to the way people are advised on managing their own dental health, through daily self-care and regular checkups).

PHASE 7: RETURN TO PLAY

Return to play is multifactorial, not only from the individual patient's perspective but also from the decision makers' perspective. In team sports, the people involved in the decision to return to play can be the doctor (who determines that the clinical evaluation shows that the patient is continuing to improve and can sustain increased load and demands of training), the scientist (who must be satisfied with the performance-related data), the fitness coach (who must be satisfied that the player has completed enough skill- and agility-related activity), and the coach (who must be satisfied that the player has completed enough training time to meet the requirements of the next game). Other stakeholders are involved with professional sport, such as the player's agent and the directors of the club. However, the most important stakeholder is the player. The player must feel ready to return to play, and this can involve a plethora of psychological and physical issues.

From a medical viewpoint, a successful return to play means that no recurrence of the injury will occur and a secondary desire that the performance of the player is as good, and possibly better, than it was before the injury (with the exception of certain aspects of the game that can only be achieved by playing the game or performing the sport in the competitive environment).

Return to play can involve reassurance from the support/rehabilitation staff that "everything will be okay," which entails disclosure of the player's success and progress to date. Psychological reassurance throughout all stages of the rehabilitation process should not be undervalued.

Occasions may arise when a player's load can be managed to enable participation. For example, a player experiencing recurrent achillodynia may be managed by being removed from the training group the day after a game. The player's first recovery day may involve training in the water, and on the second day the loading (which can be measured as stated earlier, using heart rate and GPS) can be restricted to whatever percentage the prevention team views as appropriate. The use of these modalities is in its infancy, and the reliability depends on the positioning of satellites around the world. In areas of reliable coverage, current devices are thought to be up to 15% inaccurate. These loading data should be viewed with an artistic mind at this stage, but this may become more defined in the future so that "true loading" can be matched alongside cause and effect.[33,34]

SUMMARY

Rehabilitation is easy to do badly and difficult to do well. Many people are involved in the process, and they must act as a team to support the patient with good communication and teamwork (supporting the process). A head of the rehabilitation team should be nominated, and the case manager in these circumstances should be the physician. The main practitioner performing the rehabilitation (dependent, therefore, on the stage of the process) should not be the case manager, because this person is not capable of objectively and critically evaluating the success or failure of the treatment. The case manager may most appropriately be the patient's physician. Persons or clubs without physicians may foreshorten this process; however, the consequent danger is that the failure to complete rehabilitation may result in the player seeking other expertise that may be detrimental to recovery.

The case manager must evaluate the patient on a regular basis and be involved in the decision making throughout the rehabilitation. The case manager shares information within the team and makes the decision regarding to when to progress or arrest treatment.

The whole process can be satisfying to all concerned when dealing with motivated and enthusiastic patients. Measuring the process is achievable and gives credibility and support to the initial hypothesis of the individual's rehabilitation program.

Rehabilitation involves creativity using science and art, with the end result being the patient's return to a normal life or ability to excel within their support (depending on the nature of the individual and injury).

REFERENCES

1. Della Thompson, editor. The Concise Oxford Dictionary. 9th edition. Oxford, England: Clarendon Press; 1995.
2. Waterman B, Walker JJ, Swaims C, et al. The efficacy of combined cryotherapy and compression compared with cryotherapy alone following anterior cruciate ligament reconstruction. J Knee Surg 2012;25(2):155–60.
3. Van den Bekerom MP, Struijs PA, Blankevoort L, et al. What is the evidence for rest, ice, compression, and elevation therapy in the treatment of ankle sprains in adults? J Athl Train 2012;47(4):435–43.
4. KIllgore GL. Deep water running: a practical review of the literature with an emphasis on biomechanics. Phys Sportsmed 2012;40(1):116–26.
5. Bushman BA, Flynn MG, Andrea FF, et al. Effect of 4 weeks of deep water run training on running performance. Med Sci Sports Exerc 1997;29(5):694–9.
6. DeMaere JM, Ruby BC. Effects of deep water and treadmill running on oxygen uptake and energy expenditure in seasonally trained cross country runners. J Sports Med Phys Fitness 1997;37(3):175–81.
7. Eyestone ED, Fellingham G, George J, et al. Effect of water running and cycling on maximum oxygen consumption and 2-mile run performance. Am J Sports Med 1993;21(1):41–4.
8. Killgore GL, Wilcox AR, Caster BL, et al. A lower-extremities kinematic comparison of deep-water running styles and treadmill running. J Strength Cond Res 2006;20(4):919–27.
9. Wilcox KC, Woodall WR, Stubbs PL. Development of a multifaceted aquatic exercise program for rehabilitation of athletes with patellar tendinopathy. Journal of Aquatic Physical Therapy 2007;15(2):1–9.
10. Masumoto K, Delion D, Mercer JA. Insight into muscle activity during deep water running. Med Sci Sports Exerc 2009;41(10):1958–64.
11. Mercer JA, Jensen RL. Reliability and validity of a deep water running graded exercise test. Meas Phys Educ Exerc Sci 1997;1:213–22.
12. Villalta EM, Peiris CL. Early aquatic physical therapy improves function and does not increase risk of wound-related adverse events for adults post orthopedic surgery: a systematic review and meta-analysis. Arch Phys Med Rehabil 2013;94(1):138–48.
13. The Pool Water Treatment Advisory Group. Swimming pool water. Treatment and quality standards for pools and spas. 2nd edition. 2009. ISBN0951700766.
14. Van der Wees PJ, Lenssen AF, Hendriks EJ, et al. Effectiveness of exercise therapy and manual mobilisation in ankle sprain and functional instability: a systematic review. Aust J Physiother 2006;52(1):27–37.

15. Kulig K, Popovich JM, Noceti-Dewit LM, et al. Women with posterior tibial tendon dysfunction have diminished ankle and hip muscle performance. J Orthop Sports Phys Ther 2011;41(9):687–94.
16. Palmieri RM, Ingersoll CD, Hoffman MA, et al. Arthrogenic muscle response to a simulated ankle joint effusion. Br J Sports Med 2004;38(1):26–33.
17. Holmich P, Holmich LR, Bjerg AM. Clinical examination of athletes with groin pain: an intraobserver and interobserver reliability study. Br J Sports Med 2004;38: 446–51.
18. Hölmich P, Uhrskov P, Ulniths L, et al. Effectiveness of active physical training as a treatment for long-standing adductor-related groin pain in athletes: randomised trial. Lancet 1999;353:439–43.
19. Crow J, Pearce A, Veale J, et al. Hip adductor muscle strength is reduced proceeding and during the onset of groin pain in elite junior Australian football players. J Sci Med Sport 2010;13(2):202–4.
20. Engebretsen A, Myklebust G, Holme I, et al. Intrinsic risk factors for groin injuries among male soccer players: a prospective cohort study. Am J Sports Med 2010; 38(10):2051–7.
21. Verrall G, Slavotinek J, Barnes P, et al. Description of pain provocation tests used for the diagnosis of sports-related chronic groin pain: relationship of tests to defined clinical (pain and tenderness) and MRI (pubic bone marrow oedema) criteria. Scand J Med Sci Sports 2005;15(1):36–42.
22. Bendiksen M, Ahler T, Clausen H, et al. The use of Yo-Yo IR1 and Andersen testing for fitness and maximal heart rate assessments of 6-10 yr old school children. J Strength Cond Res, in press.
23. Thomeé R, Kaplan Y, Kvist J, et al. Muscle strength and hop performance criteria prior to return to sports after ACL reconstruction. Knee Surg Sports Traumatol Arthrosc 2011;19(11):1798–805.
24. Postle K, Pak D, Smith TO. Effectiveness of proprioceptive exercises for ankle ligament injury in adults: a systematic literature and meta-analysis. Man Ther 2012;17(4):285–91.
25. Thomeé R, Neeter C, Gustavsson A, et al. Variability in leg muscle power and hop performance after anterior cruciate ligament reconstruction. Knee Surg Sports Traumatol Arthrosc 2012;20(6):1143–51.
26. Narducci E, Waltz A, Gorski K, et al. The clinical utility of functional performance tests within one year of post ACL reconstruction: a systematic review. Int J Sports Phys Ther 2011;6(4):333–42.
27. Garrison JC, Shanley E, Thigpen C, et al. The reliability of The Vail Sports Test as a measure of physical performance following anterior cruciate ligament reconstruction. Int J Sports Phys Ther 2012;7(1):20–30.
28. Kvist J. Sagittal plane knee motion in the ACL-deficient knee during body weight shift exercises on different support surfaces. J Orthop Sports Phys Ther 2006; 36(12):954–62.
29. Pinnington HC, Lloyd DG, Besier TF, et al. Kinematic and electromyography analysis of submaximal differences running on a firm surface compared with soft, dry sand. Eur J Appl Physiol 2005;94:242–53.
30. Binnie MJ, Peeling P, Pinnington H, et al. Effect of training surface on acute physiological responses following interval training. J Strength Cond Res 2013; 27(4):1047–56.
31. Aragão FA, Karamanidis K, Vaz MA, et al. Mini-trampoline exercise related to mechanisms of dynamic stability improves the ability to regain balance in elderly. J Electromyogr Kinesiol 2011;21(3):512–8.

32. Kidgell DJ, Horvath DM, Jackson BM, et al. Effect of six weeks of dura disc and mini-trampoline balance training on postural sway in athletes with functional ankle instability. J Strength Cond Res 2007;21(2):466–9.
33. Nielsen RO, Cederholm P, Buist I, et al. Can GPS be used to detect deleterious progression in training volume among runners? J Strength Cond Res, in press.
34. Scott BR, Lockie RG, Knight TJ, et al. A comparison of methods to quantify the in-season training load of professional soccer players. Int J Sports Physiol Perform 2013;8(2):195–202.

Association of Lower Limb Injury with Boot Cleat Design and Playing Surface in Elite Soccer

Anne-Marie O'Connor, DBiomechPod, DPodM, MChS, SRCh[a],
Iain T. James, PhD[b],*

KEYWORDS

- Football • Ankle sprain • Metatarsal • Natural turf • Synthetic turf • Artificial turf
- Injury • Orthotics

KEY POINTS

- Noncontact foot and ankle injury in soccer is associated with the player-boot-surface interaction.
- The mechanical properties of playing surface vary with the system (natural/synthetic turf), between clubs, between training and stadium facilities, and over the season with the effects of weather and usage.
- Boot design is surface-system and surface-condition specific and players should select their boot cleat size and configuration carefully.
- Sports medical teams should assess the specific biomechanics and physiology of players and ensure that their boot selection is appropriate and not a potential injury risk factor.

INTRODUCTION

Association football (soccer) is the highest participation global sport and a multibillion-dollar industry. The disclosed annual spend on professional player transfers in the English Premier League averaging £586 million between 2007 and 2011[1] and the direct costs (treatment and rehabilitation) and indirect costs (lost earnings and bonuses, reduced competition success) of injury are high. Therefore, keeping players injury free and performing at their peak for the 10 months of the season is very important. Foot

Dr Ian James is currrently with TGMS Ltd, Cranfield Innovation Centre, Cranfield, United Kingdom.

Disclosure: Iain James has no relationship with any commercial company that has direct financial interest in the subject matter or materials discussed in the article.

[a] Fortius Clinic, 17 Fitzhardinge Street, London W1H 6EQ, UK; [b] Centre for Sports Surface Technology, Cranfield University, Cranfield MK43 0AL, UK

* Corresponding author. TGMS Ltd, Cranfield Innovation Centre, University Way, Cranfield MK43 0BT, UK.

E-mail address: iain.james@tgms.co.uk

and particularly ankle injuries are common in football.[2] To reduce the incidence and severity of noncontact foot and ankle injuries in football requires an understanding of

1. Player condition and injury history
2. The biomechanics of the movements resulting in injury
3. The mechanics of football pitch (surface) design
4. How football boots interface with the player and the surface, and how this affects player loading

The interaction between boot and surface is critical in determining both player performance and the development of certain noncontact injuries in football. This interaction is complex, with variation in players, movement, boot design, and surface mechanical properties all determining player stability and the magnitude, direction, and rate of loading on the player. The boot is required to provide control of the player-ball interaction, protection of the foot from contact injury (contact with both other players and the playing surface), and optimum player traction. Traction is the frictional force between the boot and surface, which can be developed without slip. Insufficient traction (excessive slip) limits player speed and movement, preventing acceleration, braking, and change of direction and, therefore, has an effect on performance. Excessive traction can cause injury by fixing the players' foot to the surface and increasing both linear and angular forces on the body, which cannot be supported by the musculoskeletal system, often resulting in lower limb ligament injury in particular. Injuries to professional footballers in the United Kingdom that can be directly attributed to incorrect football boots have been estimated to cost £75 million a year.[3]

FOOT AND ANKLE INJURY IN FOOTBALL

Hawkins and colleagues[2] reported on a prospective epidemiologic study of injury in the top 4 divisions of professional football in England between July 1997 and May 1999. They observed that professional footballers are exposed to a high risk of injury, with 78% of injuries leading to a minimum of one competitive match being missed. Of the 6030 injuries reported, 17% were to the ankle and 5% to the foot, with most (67%) of these injuries occurring in competition. This finding is consistent with a range of 17% to 23% of all injuries in football being to the ankle.[4–8] Woods and colleagues[9] provided a detailed analysis of ankle injury in the same study of professional clubs. Sprain injuries formed 67% of all ankle injuries (n = 1011) whereby a player missed more than 48 hours of training. Most of these sprain injuries were to the lateral ligament complex, particularly to the anterior talofibular ligament, indicating ankle inversion as a common mechanism. Most (77%) of the noncontact injuries (39% of total ankle injuries) were during landing, twisting, turning, and running, identifying key mechanisms for the investigation of surface/boot–related injury.

The severity of ankle sprain injury was low, with 83% of players having a rehabilitation period of less than 1 month and typically missing 3 games. The analysis of severity is depends on the player and the significance of the 3 games missed, but Woods and colleagues[9] point out that it is the incidence rather than the severity of the ankle injury that is the problem in football. Effective rehabilitation was often compromised by returning to play before full ligament healing, possibly contributing to the relatively high reinjury rate, particularly in noncontact injuries.[10,11] Both studies[2,9] reported an early season bias that is common to injury epidemiology studies of football. Two causal factors have been proposed: player condition and surface hardness caused by dry summer weather conditions.[7] It is likely that this peak is related to player conditioning because it also occurs in January in elite youth football following a winter break period[4] when surfaces are likely to be in their lowest traction state because of rainfall.[12]

Modern boot design has aimed to increase player speed and stamina and increase player sensitivity when in contact with the ball by selecting lightweight materials for the sole and reducing the thickness of the upper materials to reduce the mass of the boot. This design has led to a concern that the ankle is not sufficiently supported[13] and that there is an increased risk of metatarsal injury. Coyles and Lake[14] looked at the association between stud positions and plantar pressure to explore any relationship between increased pressure caused by stud position and metatarsal fatigue. Using 3 different boots with various stud positions and analyzing player pressure distribution running on a motorized treadmill and on natural turf, they found that the pressure distribution across the forefoot was not constant between subjects for all boots analyzed. They attributed this to the variations in foot profiles and metatarsal parabola, concluding that it was not a particular boot that was at high risk of causing increased plantar pressure but rather the association between stud positions and the player's individual foot profile. Increased stud numbers, forefoot cushioning, and stiffer-soled boots along with softer playing surfaces to encourage better stud penetration were recommended to reduce this risk factor.

The design progress of football boots over recent years has aimed not only to design a lighter-weight boot but also a narrower fit to permit better sensation of the ball along the instep (reducing boot weight further). Santos and colleagues[15] investigated in-shoe dynamic foot pressures with professional footballers, looking at relationships between area, force, and pressure when comparing football boots with trainers. The plantar foot area was approximately 8% lower in the boot compared with the trainer, increasing the maximum pressure by 35%. This increased pressure is a potential increased risk factor for foot stress injuries whereby the boot is considerably narrower than the player's foot. Football is a skill-based sport with numerous repeated accelerations, decelerations, and cutting maneuvers. Players prefer minimal slip, not only with the boot-surface interface but also the foot-boot interface; to this end, players will commonly wear boots 1 to 2 (United Kingdom) sizes too small, wear double socks, or orthotics. Textured insoles have been found to increase sensory feedback and proprioception, restoring the movement discrimination back to barefoot levels when compared with the smooth insoles often found in football boots.[16] Waddington and Adams[16] recommend textured over smooth insoles as an injury prevention strategy because the plantar sole of the foot reflects changes in pressure patterns and is, therefore, an important sensor for center of pressure. A study by Percy and Menz[17] found reduced mediolateral sway when standing unipedal with prefabricated orthotics, although this orthotic did not have the textured upper described earlier, which could improve proprioception further. The authors' review did not reveal any research on the effect of insoles or orthotics in relation to shoe-surface mechanics in football.

THE ROLE OF THE SURFACE IN INJURY

Elite football matches are predominantly played on natural turf with modern long-pile, sand/rubber-filled synthetic turf used by some clubs. It is common in injury studies to categorize football pitches as simply *natural turf* or *synthetic turf*; however, this is an oversimplification.[18] Natural turf surfaces vary in construction materials and grass types but most of the elite competition pitches are constructed from freely draining sand and use perennial ryegrass (*Lolieum perenne*) or smooth stalked meadow grass (*Poa pratensis*).[19] These surfaces are often reinforced to increase wear resistance, either by the inclusion of synthetic turf fibers punched into the soil or by incorporation of fine polypropylene and rubber fibers into the sand. The shear strength (a key property in determining the hardness and traction of a playing surface) of sand is less sensitive to increases in water content than the silts and clays found in greater proportions in native soil pitches where rainfall can cause a rapid reduction in shear strength that results in loss of traction.[20] Sand-construction natural turf surfaces are more consistent temporally and spatially than native soil pitches but are also consistently harder.[12,21] The construction and maintenance costs for sand-construction pitches are high, requiring frequent application of irrigation water and fertilizer and even the use of growth lighting technology in some stadia.[19] As a consequence, these high-performance surfaces are often limited to professional stadium pitches and a small number of premiership (tier 1) training facilities. Less well-resourced clubs will have native soil stadium pitches that have greater seasonal variation in hardness and traction[12]; they are also more likely to vary in hardness and traction across the pitch,[21] which could be a greater injury risk factor. Ekstrand and Nigg[22] found 24% of lower limb football injuries were associated with poor playing surfaces and/or inferior football boots leading to excessive or insufficient traction. Where high-performance sand construction pitches are used as the main stadium pitch for competition, it is still common to find that the training pitches are native soil. This can result in differences in hardness and traction that will vary between the training and competition environment, which is not a factor considered in published football epidemiologic studies to date because of the lack of routine within-season testing of playing-surface condition.[18]

Synthetic turf surfaces can provide a more temporally and spatially consistent surface than native soil natural turf pitches. New-generation synthetic turf is different from that trialed and rejected in the 1980s at clubs, such as Oldham, Luton Town, and Queens Park Rangers. Modern synthetic turf surfaces have a longer pile length and are filled with both sand and rubber to provide a more compliant surface.[23] The risk of skin abrasion is reduced by the rubber infill and the selection of softer fiber materials, such as polypropylene. These long-pile synthetic turf surfaces are approved for use in the Union of European Football Associations and Fédération Internationale de Football Association (FIFA) competitions and several professional leagues throughout the world.[24] Although their use is prohibited for competitive matches in the English Premier League, several clubs have indoor training facilities using synthetic turf; there is currently a consultation on their use in the English Football League (tiers 2–4). In larger clubs, the indoor facilities will only be used if the players are not able to train outdoors (ie, in extreme weather conditions and snow). Having use of multiple training pitches, they are able to rotate pitches to prevent excess wear. Smaller clubs who do not have as many fields to rotate and squads who train in the evenings are more likely to use the indoor artificial surfaces; the relatively lower maintenance cost of these surfaces with higher utilization means they are more cost-effective.

It should be noted that the performance of a synthetic turf pitch also varies over space and time because of wear and compaction and that regular maintenance is required to sustain pitch performance.[25,26] Performance requirements for synthetic surfaces used in professional football are stipulated by the FIFA.[27] The premium FIFA 2-star standard requires routine testing of surface performance against several criteria that describe both the player-surface and the ball-surface interaction.

Williams and colleagues[24] analyzed 20 cohort studies and reviewed the extent to which injury patterns are different or similar between natural turf and synthetic turf surfaces. They reported strong evidence that there was only a trivial difference in injury incidence rates between modern synthetic turf and natural turf but that synthetic turf increased the risk of ankle injury in 8 out of 14 cohorts and that 6 cohorts showed that synthetic turf reduced muscle injuries in football in comparison with natural turf. They explored possible causes for the increase in ankle injury risk and reported evidence for increased traction in studies by Villwock and colleagues[28] and Livesay and colleagues.[29] The review by Williams and colleagues[24] suggested that long-term prospective cohort studies with coherent definitions of injury and severity were required. Ford and colleagues[30] compared the in-shoe plantar pressure of 17 male football players between synthetic and natural turf surfaces while performing a foot-ball-specific slalom cutting maneuver in 14-stud molded cleat boots. On synthetic turf, peak pressure was greatest central to lateral toes; however, on natural turf, maximum peak pressures were more medial and lateral forefoot. They hypothesized that the natural turf allowed the medial forefoot to sink in while cutting, which was not possible on the synthetic surface, allowing the foot to invert. These higher peak forces will be increased further with increased mass or acceleration in a game situation; this increased plantar force and, thus, frictional resistance is potentially injurious.[31]

Currently, there is a discrepancy between training surfaces and stadium competition surfaces, whether training on synthetic or natural turf. Larger clubs ensure that training pitches are of similar size and construction to stadium pitches, but there are large associated construction and maintenance costs. Smaller clubs will be training on surfaces that are different from their competition pitches. There is a need for a large-scale investigation of how and whether competition injuries relate to the contrast between training and competition surface conditions, acknowledging that there will be variation when competing at away fixtures. The advantage of using high-quality artificial surfaces (new third-generation turf [3G]) in stadiums and playing fields is principally reduced operating costs, but there is also the potential to create the same surface and traction in all stadiums and pitches year round.

MEASURING SURFACE PROPERTIES

Measurements of the surface impact response and traction aim to provide insight into the player-boot-surface interaction. The devices used to measure these properties vary in their complexity and relevance to actual boundary conditions of loading rate, magnitude, and orientation.[32,33] Devices for characterizing surface impact response include the penetrometer, the Clegg Impact Surface Tester (CIST [SD Instrumentation, Bath, UK]), and the Artificial Athlete (AA [Deltec Equipment, Duiven, The Netherlands]). Orchard[34] used a penetrometer to measure the hardness of the ground in the Australian Football League throughout a season and found that the ground was hardest at the beginning few months and softened up as the season progressed; he also found that the incidences of anterior cruciate ligament (ACL) injuries reduced as the season progressed and the ground became softer. The penetrometer provides an indication of the penetration hardness of a surface. High penetration resistance can prevent full cleat penetration of the surface by the boot, preventing load distribution across the whole sole or area of the sole in contact with the surface, leading to stress localizations in the foot above the cleats.[33] Such conditions can exist on clay soil pitches during the summer; a range of strategies can be used to prevent related injuries, such as pitch watering or the use of shorter cleats or molded-rubber clear-soled boots. The CIST uses an accelerometer within a cylindrical mass (typically 2.25 kg) that is dropped from a specific height (typically 0.45 m) to determine peak deceleration on impact (in multiples of the acceleration caused by gravity); greater rebound hardness results in increased peak deceleration. In a study of natural turf,[12] it was shown that the penetrometer and the CIST are correlated; but neither device is representative of the magnitude or rate of loading applied by players performing sports-specific movements. For example, Caple and colleagues[35] showed that the CIST (2.25 kg) applied a peak vertical stress of 600 kN m^{-2} with a loading duration of 8.2 milliseconds; the peak stress for an 80-kg human running on natural turf at 3.8 ms^{-1} was 553 kN m^{-2} but the duration of loading was 120 milliseconds. The mechanical behavior of sport surfaces is rate dependent[36]; therefore, the loading rate is important. The AA is designed to apply the load over a greater period by using a spring of known stiffness to attenuate a falling mass. The device measures the force reduction of a surface relative to concrete. More advanced variants can also determine energy restitution using an accelerometer.[23] Force reduction measurement is a key component of the FIFA approval system for synthetic turf surfaces.[27]

Traction is commonly split into 2 types: linear and rotational. Linear traction is measured by fixing cleats to a weighted sled that is moved horizontally over the surface at a range of normal loads using mechanical, electromechanical, or pneumatic systems.[37] Alternatively, linear traction can be measured using a pendulum device, although this is increasingly rare. Rotational traction is most commonly measured using a weighted studded disc that is dropped onto the surface to aid stud penetration and then rotated and a peak torque is measured. This example is one of a fixed rate, fixed orientation device that is suitable for comparing one surface with another; however, Kirk and colleagues[33] identified that limiting stud configuration, stud/sole orientation with respect to the surface, and load magnitude/rate does not provide realistic boundary conditions for actual player movement and, therefore, injury mechanism. In reality, player-boot-surface interaction in a single movement involves a range of loading directions, rotation of forces through the movement, and a change in the contact area and the orientation of the boot.[19,33] Measurements of peak torque and peak linear resistance are considered an oversimplification of the player-surface interaction, and the investigation of surface behavior is more reliably informed by considering the whole force-displacement/torque-rotation curve[23,33,38] and particularly when the boot first starts to move because peak resistance can occur at displacements much larger than that exhibited during real player-surface interaction.[33,37]

To understand injury mechanism there is a need for more biomechanically valid testing devices; however, there is a trade-off between device complexity and the cost and portability of testing devices, which results in limited use of more complex devices.[32] Prospective epidemiologic studies of injury in football would benefit from valid, parallel, routine characterization of surface type, hardness, and traction in addition to standardized injury reporting. Simply designating the surface as natural or synthetic ignores the variation in system types that exists within these categories.[18,19,23]

BOOT DESIGN AND SELECTION STRATEGY FOR REDUCED INJURY RISK

There is a range of boot design factors that affect traction, including sole shape and features, cleat shape, cleat length, and cleat arrangement.[39] Boot manufacturers can vary these factors to optimize traction for maximum performance and minimum injury risk. With surface mechanical properties that change through space and time across a pitch and between pitches of different construction types, optimum boot design is expected to vary; therefore, players could require a range of boot designs depending on the range of surface conditions they can expect to encounter.

For elite players, particularly internationals, boot selection is related to commercial contracts with a single manufacturer. The football boot manufacturers who sponsor players have a vested interest in keeping their players injury free because the players are wearing and advertising their boots on a world stage. The manufacturers are regularly in contact with their sponsored players for their feedback on boot construction, including traction, comfort, performance, and aesthetics; they use this feedback in their future designs. Most often the sponsored player will be given a regular boot and then the manufacturer will customize it to the player's needs, with additional padding for comfort, stretching for toe deformities, and embroidery requested by the player (eg, the flag of their country or their name). Alternatively, if the player is not compatible with the over-the-counter boot, the sponsor usually has facilities to create a customized boot with a last of the player's foot, created to the needs of the individual; this process is more costly.

Boot manufacturers are also becoming more interested in liaising with the clubs medical team, acknowledging they have a very important role to play in both the prevention and rehabilitation of player foot and ankle injuries. Example instructions from the medical team could include the following: modifying boots to provide extra stability for a recovering metatarsal fracture, Lisfranc disruption or problematic sesamoid, alteration of the boot heel tab for an Achilles tendon or retrocalcaneal exostosis, or extra height along the sole plate for a leg-length discrepancy. Boot alteration is an important consideration for player foot rehabilitation and earlier return to play. Achieving such modifications with nonsponsored players in lower tiers of competition is a challenge and requires specialist adaptation services.

Traditionally, football boot cleats were conical; but in 1996, the first elongated cleat (or blade) was made commercially available. The bladed cleat has an increased surface area of contact compared with the conical cleat and is designed to increase traction and reduce slip. However, the shape is nonsymmetric; therefore, resistance varies with the orientation of loading. This design has been adopted by a range of manufacturers who have sought to optimize cleat shape and configuration below the foot, with some manufacturers individually designing each cleat position and shape for a specific function. Generally, boots are available in 3 configurations that decrease the number of studs but increase the length of studs because surfaces offer lower traction: artificial turf (AG/TG) with numerous short cleats or a pimpled rubber sole; firm ground (FG) with relatively short, bladed cleats; and soft ground (SG), with longer, interchangeable studs to provide greater traction. It is important that players match the boot type to the surface type/condition. Müller and colleagues[40] investigated the effect of boot sole type with increasing stud length (zero stud, AG, FG, and SG) on lower limb kinematics and kinetics during a 135° turning movement on third-generation synthetic turf. They observed that in the zero-stud treatment, players kept shank alignment more vertical to limit horizontal forces and slip. The SG design, not normally used on synthetic turf because of the excessive stud length and traction, reduced mediolateral foot translation (horizontal slip), increased ankle moments, and was implied to increase loading on the body when used on an inappropriate surface.

Fig. 1 shows a range of modern FG boots, with a variety of stud shapes and configurations. Some boots have the cleats on the forefoot placed in a linear shape around the peripheral edge (see **Fig. 1**A), and some are more curved around the peripheral and central forefoot cleats varying in numbers from 1 to 2 (see **Fig. 1**B–D). The shape of the cleats also vary, either being wedge shaped, oval, triangular, or conical (see **Fig. 1**).

The adoption of blade instead of conical cleats has generated considerable debate within the sport and in the literature. Lambson and colleagues[41] looked at the correlation between ACL injuries and 4 football boots with different cleat designs, concluding that the boot with blades shaped peripherally and with longer cleats significantly increased the shoe-surface traction and, therefore, put the player at an increased risk of developing ACL injuries. They also tested all 4 boots both on grass

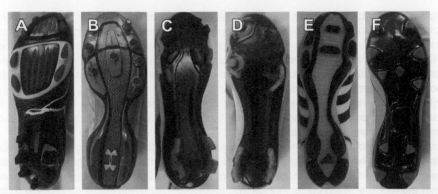

Fig. 1. Different cleat shape, size, and configuration in (A) Puma Powercat FG (Puma SE, Herzogenaurach, Germany), (B) Under Armour Dominate FG (Under Armour Inc, Baltimore, MD), (C) Nike Vapor FG (Nike Inc, Beaverton, OR), (D) Nike Mercurial Vapor, (E) Adidas Adi-Pure FG (Adidas AG, Herzogenaurach, Germany), (F) Adidas F50 FG.

and sand-filled, short-pile synthetic turf surfaces and consistently found increased torsion resistance with the synthetic turf. Scranton and colleagues[42] studied noncontact ACL injuries in American football and found there was a lower incidence of ACL injuries with players who used spatting taping techniques (taping over the ankle and the outside of the boot). It was hypothesized that using this particular taping technique, because it passes over the studs, will effectively reduce their penetration into the playing surface and, hence, reduce traction. Kaila[43] studied knee loading when performing a side-step cutting maneuver comparing 2 different conical cleat boots and 2 different bladed boots. He concluded that the knee valgus angle was the same for all 4 boots in each trial but raised a concern that side-step cutting significantly increased internal tibial and valgus moments and anterior joint forces, which could be implicated in noncontact ACL injuries. Bentley and colleagues[44] compared plantar pressure distribution between the same boot with conical and bladed cleats. Their studies included 29 amateur football players running in a straight line and slalom on long-pile synthetic turf. They found significant differences between forefoot loading between the two boots, with more pressure distribution on the medial aspect of the conical cleat boot and the lateral aspect of the bladed boot. They concluded that the conical studded boot was safer because it mimics a normal motif and deemed the bladed boot as potentially harmful because of the unnatural increase in lateral foot loading.

DISCUSSION

There is an association of lower limb injuries with boot cleat design and playing surfaces.[3,7,13,15,27–29] There is a need in soccer to control the external injury risk factors of boots and surfaces both separately and their interaction during the course of play. In theory, standardization of these external risk factors would be an obvious solution to injury prevention. But it is difficult to standardize playing surfaces throughout the soccer leagues or even within the same division (tier) because of the variations in construction and age of each club's natural and synthetic turfs discussed earlier. Standardizing boot cleat configuration is also difficult because of the commercial behavior of manufacturers who need to create new, unique designs and also because of a player's individual choice and biomechanics. Some manufacturers will change sole and cleat configuration annually, making it difficult for researchers to investigate the effect each boot has on foot pressures and the boot-surface interaction.

The choice of boot is generally very player and position specific. The lower-mass highly skilled striker and attacking midfielder may prefer lighter-weight performance boots with higher traction for sharper accelerations, decelerations, and side stepping. Higher-mass central defenders and goal keepers may choose a more robust boot for greater kicking power and a padded upper for foot protection against contact injuries from other players, such as deliberate stamping during set-piece moves. Boot sponsorship agreements between manufacturers and players play a significant role in determining footwear selection and generally dictate that the player wears only one design of their brand for all competitions and training; but occasionally, the international players are required to wear a particular boot for domestic competitions and a different design of the same brand for international games or European club competition games in an attempt to reach an alternative viewing audience. This situation makes familiarity of the player with the boot and surface more difficult. Standardizing cleat configuration is also difficult because each player's foot profile is unique to them and they will, therefore, respond in different ways to boot-cleat plantar pressure[13]; therefore, the best boot for one player is not necessarily the best boot for another. In addition, cleat/foot pressure and their interaction with the surface will vary because of player mass, speed, and style of play; for example, traction on rotation will vary with the same boot on different players.[30]

A player is more likely to suffer a lower limb injury as a result of the boot cleat design and playing surface if the player has less-than-optimal conditioning, has a previous lower limb injury history, and their style of play involves numerous rotations on the surface. External risk factors increase the risk, such as less-than-optimum surface design/condition, a boot style or cleat design that is not best suited to the players foot profile, or a surface that has less-than-optimum traction with the cleats.

SUMMARY

To reduce risk factors for foot and ankle injury, elite players should be assessed by the club medical team to ensure that they are wearing the most suitable boot for their foot profile; to liaise with their sponsor when necessary, especially if they have had a previous foot or lower limb injury; and to modify their boots or provide appropriate insoles or orthotics. The mechanical properties of playing surfaces are not standardized across clubs within a competition, and even within the same club there can be significant differences in training pitches and match pitches. These pitches will vary over space and time because of weather and wear factors. Players should be educated to select boots according to (1) surface type and (2) surface condition (ie, it is not enough to match artificial turf [AT] boots to artificial surfaces and soft ground [SG] boots to natural turf); even within the same surface type, the surface properties will change from venue to venue and from month to month depending on the weather and any irrigation applied. To inform coaches and players of surface conditions and cleat selection would require a level of routine pitch testing that is not currently adopted in professional football. The referee routinely checks the cleats of players' boots before entering the field of play, but this is to ensure that they are not sharp enough to cause injury to another player; there is no feedback on the safety of the boots for the player wearing them. Ideally, a portable device would be available to measure the surface impact response and the linear and rotation traction with the latest boot cleat designs, along with providing optimum guidelines.[45] This testing could be done by grounds staff and the surface watered appropriately to alter surface traction or advice given to players regarding the most suitable boot for surface conditions.

Research into the effects of boot design, particularly the cleat shape and configuration, is at an early stage; commercial evolution in boot design is fast paced. As a consequence, there is only a small body of evidence available on the interaction between football boot design, surface type, and the properties of the surface at the point of injury. On presentation of foot or ankle injuries, the medical team should determine whether the surface type, surface condition, boot type, boot width, and cleat configuration are critical factors when considering the injury mechanism and how this relates to the patients' injury history.

REFERENCES

1. Deloitte. Premier League clubs' transfer spending cut. United Kingdom: Sport Business Group, Deloitte LLP. Available at: http://www.deloitte.com/view/en_GB/uk/industries/sportsbusinessgroup/ebdd7dcf77835310VgnVCM3000001c56f00aRCRD.htm. Accessed April 20, 2012.
2. Hawkins RD, Hulse MA, Wilkinson C, et al. The association football medical research programme: an audit of injuries in professional football. Br J Sports Med 2001;35:43–7.
3. Morag E. Recent advancements in football equipment design for youth and adult players. 'The medical field; a Nike Sports research review', vol. 9. Beaverton (OR): Nike, Inc; 2003. p. 1.
4. Cloke DJ, Spencer S, Hodson A, et al. The epidemiology of ankle injuries occurring in English football academies. Br J Sports Med 2009;43:1119–25.
5. Hawkins RD, Fuller CW. A prospective epidemiological study of injuries in for English professional football clubs. Br J Sports Med 1999;33:196–203.
6. LeGall F, Carling C, Reilly T, et al. Incidence of injuries in elite French youth soccer players: a 10-season study. Am J Sports Med 2006;34:928–38.
7. Price RJ, Hawkins RD, Hulse MA, et al. The Football Association medical research programme: an audit of injuries in academy youth football. Br J Sports Med 2004;38:466–71.
8. Schmidt-Olsen S, Jorgensen U, Kallund S, et al. Injuries among young soccer players. Am J Sports Med 1991;19:273–5.
9. Woods C, Hawkins R, Hulse M, et al. The Football Association medical research programme: an audit of injuries in professional football: an analysis of ankle sprains. Br J Sports Med 2003;37:233–8.
10. Nielsen AB, Yde J. Epidemiology and traumatology of injuries in soccer. Am J Sports Med 1989;17:803–7.
11. Ekstrand J, Gillquist J. The avoidability of soccer injuries. Int J Sports Med 1983; 2:120–8.
12. Caple MC, James IT, Bartlett MD. Mechanical behaviour of natural turf sports pitches across a season. Sports Eng 2012;15:129–41.
13. Lees A, Nolan L. The biomechanics of soccer: a review. J Sports Sci 1998;16: 211–34.
14. Coyles VR, Lake MJ. Forefoot plantar pressure distribution inside the soccer boot during running. In: Hennig EM, Stefanyshin DJ, editors. Proceedings of the Fourth Symposium on Footwear Biomechanics. Canmore, Calgary (Canada): University of Calgary; 1999. p. 30–1.
15. Santos D, Carline T, Flynn L, et al. Distribution of in-shoe dynamic plantar foot pressures in professional football players. Foot 2001;11:10–4.

16. Waddinton G, Adams R. Football boot insoles and sensitivity to extent of ankle inversion movement. Br J Sports Med 2003;37:170–5.
17. Percy ML, Menz HB. Effects of prefabricated foot orthoses and soft insoles on postural stability in professional soccer players. J Am Podiatr Med Assoc 2001; 91:194–203.
18. Stiles VH, James IT, Dixon SJ, et al. Natural turf surfaces the case for continued research. Sports Med 2009;39:65–84.
19. James IT. Advancing natural turf to meet tomorrow's challenges. Proc Inst Mech Eng P J Sports Eng Tech 2011;225(P):115–29.
20. Guisasola I, James I, Llewellyn C, et al. Quasi-static mechanical behaviour of soils used for natural turf sports surfaces and stud force prediction. Sports Eng 2010;12:99–109.
21. Caple MC, James IT, Bartlett MD. Spatial analysis of the mechanical behaviour of natural turf sports pitches. Sports Eng 2012;15:143–57.
22. Ekstrand J, Nigg BM. Surface-related injuries in soccer. Sports Med 1989;8: 56–62.
23. Fleming P. Artificial turf systems for sports surfaces: current knowledge and research needs. Proc Inst Mech Eng P J Sports Eng Tech 2011;225:43–64.
24. Williams S, Hume PA, Kara S. A review of football injuries on third and fourth generation artificial turfs compared with natural turf. Sports Med 2011;41:903–23.
25. James IT, McLeod AJ. The effect of maintenance on the performance of sand-filled synthetic turf surfaces. Sports Tech 2010;3:43–51.
26. Fleming P. Maintenance best practice and recent research. Proc Inst Mech Eng P J Sports Eng Tech 2011;225:159–70.
27. FIFA. Quality concept for football turf. edition. Zurich (Switzerland): Fédération Internationale de Football Association (FIFA); 2012. Available at: http://www.fifa.com/mm/document/footballdevelopment/footballturf/01/13/56/08/fqchandbookof requirements(january2012).pdf. Accessed April 23, 2012.
28. Villwock MR, Meyer EG, Powell JW, et al. Football playing surface and shoe design affect rotational traction. Am J Sports Med 2009;37:518–25.
29. Livesay GA, Reda DR, Nauman EA. Peak torque and rotational stiffness developed at the shoe-surface interface: the effect of shoe type and playing surface. Am J Sports Med 2006;34:415–22.
30. Ford KR, Manson NA, Evans BJ, et al. Comparison of in-shoe foot loading patterns on natural grass and synthetic turf. J Sci Med Sport 2006;9:433–40.
31. Crawley PW, Heidt RS, Scranton PE, et al. Physiological axial load, frictional resistance, and football shoe-surface interface. Foot Ankle Int 2003;24:551–6.
32. Bartlett MD, James IT, Ford M, et al. Testing natural turf sports surfaces: the value of performance quality standards. Proc Inst Mech Eng P J Sports Eng Tech 2009; 223:21–9.
33. Kirk RF, Noble IS, Mitchell T, et al. High-speed observation of football-boot-surface interaction of players in their natural environment. Sports Eng 2007;10:129–44.
34. Orchard J. The AFL penetrometer study; work in progress. J Sci Med Sport 2001; 4:220–32.
35. Caple MC, James IT, Bartlett MD. The effect of grass leaf height on the impact behaviour of natural turf sports field surfaces. Sports Tech 2011;4:29–40.
36. Guisasola I, James I, Stiles V, et al. Dynamic behaviour of soils used for natural turf sports surfaces. Sports Eng 2010;12:111–2.
37. Severn KA, Fleming PR, Clarke JD, et al. Science of synthetic turf surfaces: investigating traction behaviour. Proc Inst Mech Eng P J Sports Eng Tech 2011;225: 147–58.

38. Fujikake K, Yamamoto T, Takemura M. A comparison of the mechanical charac-
    teristics of natural turf and artificial turf football pitches. Football Science 2007;
    4:1–8. Available at: http://www.shobix.co.jp/jssf/tempfiles/journal/2007/012.pdf.
39. Kirk B, Carré M, Haake S, et al. Modelling traction of studded footwear on sports
    surfaces using neural networks. In: Moritz EF, Haake S, editors. The engineering
    of sport 6: volume 3 developments for innovation. New York: Springer; 2006.
    p. 403–8.
40. Müller C, Sterzing T, Lake M, et al. Different stud configurations cause movement
    adaptations during a soccer turning movement. Footwear Sci 2010;2:21–8.
41. Lambson RB, Barnhill BS, Higgins RW. Football cleat design and its effect on
    anterior cruciate ligament injuries: a three-year prospective study. Am J Sports
    Med 1996;24:155–9.
42. Scranton PE, Whitesel JP, Powell JW, et al. A review of selected noncontact ante-
    rior cruciate ligament injuries in the National Football League. Foot Ankle Int 1997;
    18:772–6.
43. Kaila R. Influence of modern studded and bladed soccer boots and sidestep
    cutting on knee loading during match play conditions. Am J Sports Med 2007;
    35:1528–36.
44. Bentley JA, Ramanathan AK, Arnold GP, et al. Harmful cleats of football boots:
    a biomechanical evaluation. Foot Ankle Surg 2011;17:140–4.
45. Caple MC, James IT, Bartlett MD. Using the GoingStick to assess pitch quality.
    Proc Inst Mech Eng P J Sports Eng Tech 2012. http://dx.doi.org/10.1177/
    1754337112447268.

Index

A

Foot Ankle Clin N Am 18 (2013) 381–409
http://dx.doi.org/10.1016/S1083-7515(13)00036-3
1083-7515/13/$ – see front matter © 2013 Elsevier Inc. All rights reserved.

foot.theclinics.com

Printed and bound by CPI Group (UK) Ltd, Croydon, CR0 4YY

03/10/2024

01040440-0004